COMPLETE CANCER DIET COOKBOOK AND GUIDE

Starve the Cancer Without Starving Yourself and Win the Fight – Healthy, Tasty, and Nourishing Recipes for Cancer Treatment and Recovery!

AUGUST HARSON

TABLE OF CONTENTS

Introduction 5
Cancer Prevention and Food Preparation Suggestions 10
Foods to Try 14
Avoided Foods 17
Breakfast 19
    French Toast with Stuffing 19
    Florentine English Muffins with Egg Whites 19
    Florentine eggs 21
    Burrito for Breakfast 22
    Omelet Veggie Egg White 23
    Serves 2 24
    Pizza for Breakfast 24
    Pancakes with Cornmeal 26
    Compote de fruits frais 27
    Green Omelette 28
    Scrambled Eggs with Indian Spices 29
    Casserole with Hash Browns and Eggs 30
    Pancakes with Oatmeal 32
    Hot Cereal with Whole Grain 33
    Pancakes with Ricotta and Blueberries 33
    French Toast with Stuffing 35
Snacks and Smoothies 38
    Smoothie with Pineapple, Banana, and Cacao 38
    Smoothie with Almond Butter 38
    Smoothie with apricots and pineapples 39
    Smoothie with Mango 39
    Smoothie with Bananas and Oranges 40
    Smoothie with Berries 41
    Smoothie with Pineapple, Banana, and Cacao 41
    Smoothie with Kale 42
    Garbanzo Beans, Roasted 43
    Smoothie with peaches 44

  Trail Mix is a healthy snack. 44
Bread - Cornbread 46
  Irish Soda Bread (Whole Wheat) 46
  Muffins with apples, carrots, and raisins 47
  Banana Cinnamon Bread 48
  Ciabatta Baguette 50
  Coffee Cake with Poppy Seeds and Citrus 51
  Cornbread 52
  Bread with Garlic 53
  Whole Wheat Bread, Plain 53
  Garlic Flatbread That Isn't So Flat 55
  Bread with Herbs 56
  Pumpkin Bread with Oatmeal Topping 58
  Topping for Oatmeal 59
  Oatmeal Topping on Sweet Potato Bread 60
  Blueberry Muffins Made with Whole Wheat 61
  Irish Soda Bread (Whole Wheat) 62
  Pita Bread (Whole Wheat) 63
  Bread with Zucchini 64
  Bread with Cinnamon and Raisins 65
Sandwiches 68
  Panini with Roasted Vegetables 68
  Fries and cheeseburger 68
  Wraps made from lavash 69
  Burgers with Portobello Mushrooms 70
  Burgers with Mushrooms and Veggies 71
  Panini with Onion and Pepper 72
  Panini with Roasted Vegetables 74
  Pita Bread Salad 75
  Burgers with salmon 76
Salads 78
  Coleslaw with Indian Spices 78
  Marinated Tomatoes, Arugula, and Mushrooms 78
  Salad with Asparagus and Tomatoes 79

Salad Toppings with Avocado and Tomatoes 80
Salad with Brown Rice and Curry 81
Salad with Barley and Vegetables 82
Salad with beets 83
Salad with Carrots and Raisins 85
Slaw with Cole Slaw 86
Salad with Citrus and Ginger Dressing 87
Salad with Chops 88
Salad with White Eggs 89
Salad with Fennel 90
Cole Slaw with Indian Spices 91
Salad with potatoes 92
Salad with Kale, Tomatoes, and Avocado 94
Tomatoes Marinated 95
Salad with Roasted Broccoli 95
Salad with Spinach, Mushrooms, and Grilled Onions 96
Salad with Roasted Corn 97
Salad with Roasted Vegetables 98
Salad with salmon 100

Pizzas 102
Pizza with Garlic Salad 102
Pizza Crust Made with Whole Wheat 102
Sauce for Pizza 104
Pizza with Garlic Salad 104
Pizza with Grilled Asparagus and Mushrooms 106
Pizza with Tomato and Basil 107
Pizza from Mexico 108
Pizza with Pesto 110
Pizza with Sautéed Peppers and Onions 111
Pizza with Roasted Vegetables 112

INTRODUCTION

My doctor told me in the summer of 2004 that I had late-stage cancer and that I had a 15% chance of survival. I knew there wasn't much I could do about my cancer journey, but I was determined to make the most of what I could, namely nutrition and exercise. I immediately began a long-term study effort on foods and their links to cancer. I discovered the following: Some foods have been scientifically shown to help avoid certain cancers, while others have been proven to help cause specific cancers. Specific diet has been proven in studies to help prevent cancers, but not for other cancers...yet. So to yet, the evidence for certain malignancies is unclear, but that does not rule out the possibility that it may prove positive at some point in the future. In the meanwhile, it is acceptable to eat as healthily as possible.

You've undoubtedly picked up this book because you have cancer or know someone who does. To be honest, who doesn't? The American Cancer Society claims that

Cancer is the umbrella term for collecting more than 100 illnesses in which cells in a specific area of the body begin to proliferate uncontrollably. Although we try to ignore it as we go about our daily lives, it is, in reality, an epidemic. We ignore it and walk around it like an elephant in the centre of the room until we are forced to deal with it. We believe that if we ignore it, it will go away. Cancer remains the feared "C" word. Everyone is scared to speak or discuss it. Unfortunately, it isn't going away. The elephant is just growing in size. I hear that all the time: my mother, sister, father-in-law, kid, dog... This creature has no defences. It will ultimately affect every one of us in some manner.

Nonetheless, we keep tiptoeing around it, thinking it will not happen to us, but it may. When they get a scary diagnosis, most individuals will try everything to help themselves. Why not start now, before you have to go through what I went through? Do you want your children to have to go through what I went through?

According to recent research, if you are a woman reading this book, you have one in three risks of developing cancer in your lifetime., not your neighbour or coworker. So don't expect it to constantly be someone else. The truth is that you have a decent probability of obtaining it. It's much worse if you're a man or a baby. You have a one-in-two chance of winning. Children born today have a dreadful 50/50 chance of developing cancer in their lives unless changes are done.

There is some light amid the gloom here. According to a report published in the online journal Cancer (March 2012), the United States Centers for Disease Control and Prevention, the American Cancer Society, the National Cancer Institute, and the North American Association of Central Cancer Registries reported that death rates for all cancers, including the four most common (lung, colorectal, breast, and prostate), have steadily declined from 1999 to 2008. The decrease in cancer fatalities and new cases is thought to be due to improved scientific knowledge of how to detect, treat, and prevent cancer in the first place.

That is not to say we are powerless in the face of it. Especially if we begin now, before the dreadful diagnosis when we are still in good condition. Cancer is no longer thought to be a random occurrence or to be mainly caused by heredity. In reality, only a tiny percentage of all malignancies are caused by genetic predispositions from our forefathers. Many cancers are caused by environmental factors, poor nutrition, and a lack of activity. Research performed by the University of Copenhagen and published in the New England Journal of Medicine in March 1988 found that infants adopted at birth had similar early death rates (including cancer) to their adoptive parents. There was no link found between infant death rates and birth parents.

You may be saying to yourself, "Who are you to advise me how to avoid cancer?" You've got it! That's true, I did, but I didn't get it back when the odds were stacked against me—and I think it was my diet and exercise regimen that kept it from happening again. Unfortunately, at this moment, scientific evidence is unclear as to whether nutrition may substantially aid in preventing cancer recurrence. Nonetheless, the American Cancer Society has published suggested recommendations for cancer survivors to maintain a healthy lifestyle. They have long advocated these measures to help avoid specific malignancies, but they now propose the same standards for cancer survivors to help prevent cancer recurrence.

Their advice is to avoid cigarettes, keep a healthy weight, exercise, minimize sitting time, and consume fruits, vegetables, and whole grains. They also advise reducing your consumption of red meat, processed meat, and alcohol. These are the same recommendations I make in my eating plan.

Because there is substantial evidence that a plant-based diet reduces cancer risk overall, I decided to err on the side of caution, and the American Cancer Society now agrees. Therefore, I decided to design and follow a diet focused on foods proven to help prevent cancer, even though scientific studies on their efficacy in recurrence prevention were still ongoing.

The truth is that we don't know why some people develop cancer and others don't or why the time is so critical. Meanwhile, it stands to reason that maintaining your body as healthy as possible, including before, through, and after the cancer process, helps in the battle against the illness. For example, although scientific evidence is still developing, I think that eating a fresh salad is healthier for your body and more cancer-preventative than a glazed doughnut.

Years ago, I buried my head in the sand, believing that cancer was something that happened to other people, not to me. I was in my forties and somewhat overweight. I didn't eat horribly, but my diet wasn't great either. I didn't exercise much and was under a lot of stress in my life. I was constantly up to date on which foods were harmful to me and which were healthy for me, but to be honest, everything went in one ear and out the other. What will they tell me is terrible for me next? Blah, blah, blah. I went through life blissfully eating whatever I pleased, purchasing larger-sized clothes as middle age crept up, always thinking the Big C would not knock on my door. Looking back, it was just a question of time for me.

My first (incorrect) early cancer diagnosis was lymphoma; since the disease had spread to so many lymph nodes, it appeared as lymphoma. Following further testing, I was diagnosed with late-stage fallopian tube cancer. My doctor indicated that I only had a 15% chance of life. Six months later, following standard therapy, I cured the illness (as many women do). My doctor then estimated that there was a 75% probability of a recurrence. That is why late-stage ovarian/fallopian tube cancer is so deadly. You can get clean from it, but remaining clean is almost difficult. It is fairly uncommon for women to be cancer-free after being diagnosed with this illness. It is rare to be cancer-free for so long.

Because of the high recurrence incidence of ovarian/fallopian tube cancer during the first three years, pharmaceutical firms are developing medicines to prevent recurrences. I participated in a clinical study for one of these promising medicines held in hospitals throughout the nation. Unfortunately, the trial was terminated after nine months because it was apparent that the medication was not working—too many of the women in the study had relapsed. I was the only lady in my hospital's trial who hadn't.

One online buddy who was also a participant in the scientific study once told me, "Oh, I could never give up meat." I'd die if I had to stop eating beef. What she should have said was, "I'm going to die if I don't give up meat." But she didn't, and then she did. So I am aware that I have been granted a second shot at life. I was and continue to be cancer-free after literally years of dietary study and living the walk. There has never been a recurrence for me.

There is a lot of scientific evidence that eating properly may help prevent cancer, and eating wrong can help cause cancer. Although scientific data is still divided, and research on foods that prevent recurrence is ongoing, I feel that my diet and lifestyle keep me cancer-free. Even though the odds were stacked against me, here I am, feeling as good as or better than I did in my twenties. Scientific data shows that a healthy diet and regular exercise may substantially decrease the risk of developing cancer in the first place.

Eating, of course, must be a pleasant sensory experience and a healthy one for the body. So I set out to write a cookbook full of tasty dishes that would appeal to those who enjoyed eating excellent food rather than a health food book. I wrote a cookbook using ordinary foods for everyday families since not everyone has the time or money to go to health food shops or farmer's markets, yet everyone is at risk of getting cancer.

I've always like eating, and I've always enjoyed cooking! I'm a bit of pro—I've spent a long time in the restaurant industry, owning, managing, and cooking. Eating, and I am longtime friends. I've reorganized my kitchen and my life to focus on cancer prevention. You can, too, with a little effort.

CANCER PREVENTION AND FOOD PREPARATION SUGGESTIONS

I stay away from artificial sweeteners. Although preliminary research on several of them has indicated that they induce cancer in rats, further research has shown that they do not cause cancer in people. Studies are still ongoing, and I don't want to take any chances. We are used to consuming excessively sugary meals, particularly in our nation. I try to eat organically and have become used to (and now like) meals that are not too sweet. So what's the point of taking a chance? Who knows what the results of the next research will be?

Garlic contains many compounds that have been and continue to be investigated for their anti-cancer properties. Cooked garlic, on the other hand, has been found to lose its potential cancer-fighting qualities. Begin by crushing, mincing, or chopping your garlic before proceeding with the remainder of the dish preparation. Allowing crushed garlic to sit for even 10 minutes allows the garlic to retain its potential anti-cancer effects throughout cooking.

Grilling and lighting up the grill is something we all enjoy doing. Cooking meats at high heat, on the other hand, produces carcinogenic chemicals known as HCAs (heterocyclic amines). HCAs have been linked to cancer. This is true not just for red meat but also for chicken and fish. Fruits and vegetables, on the other hand, do not generate HCAs. So grill your fruits and vegetables to your heart's delight, but avoid grilling meats. However, if you insist on throwing meat on the grill, here are some grilling safety precautions that can lower your cancer risk:

Avoid flare-ups from fat dripping on the grill by doing the following:

- Using leaner cuts of meat or seafood.

- Keeping a spray bottle filled with water near the grill and dousing flare-ups as they occur.

- Place the meat/fish on a piece of foil with a few holes

punched in it rather than straight on the grill.

- Making use of a marinade. Marinating meat or fish before grilling has been proven to significantly decrease HCA generation.

- Avoiding charring or scorching the meat (often, turning the meat/fish helps).

- Cooking time is reduced by using a lesser amount.

- Prepare the meat for grilling by par-cooking it.

- Maintaining a low-heat setting on the grill.

Onions have been proven to help prevent cancer, but new research goes one step further: the stronger smelling onions contain more antioxidants than the softer tasting ones. Shallots, Western Yellow, New York Bold, and Northern Red have a greater flavour and better antioxidant levels. On the other hand, Empire Sweet, Western White, Peruvian Sweet, Mexico, Texas 1015, Imperial Valley Sweet, and Vidalia are sweeter and contain fewer antioxidants.

The percentage of unsaturated and saturated fats in oils varies significantly. I usually use olive and canola oils since they are rich in unsaturated fats and low in saturated fats.

Pesticides should be avoided since some have been proven to cause cancer. In addition, pesticide workers are more likely to get certain malignancies.

Physical activity and regular exercise are essential for maintaining good health. The most recent guideline is 30 minutes of moderate to intense activity each day. Walking and biking are examples of moderate exercise. Swimming and racing are examples of intense exercise. The conversation test is a solid rule of thumb. You are exercising at a moderate level if you can speak properly but not sing. You are exercising vigorously if you can only speak a few words without taking a breath. Make it a habit to work out with a friend.

Salads are delicious but skip the iceberg lettuce. Most restaurants now offer iceberg lettuce, although it is mainly water and has little nutritional benefit. Instead, use hearty greens like arugula, cabbage, spinach, kale, collard greens, mustard greens, or watercress.

Tobacco use should be avoided at all costs. According to the National Cancer Institute, tobacco smoke contains over 7,000 compounds, at least 250 of which are known to be hazardous. 69 of the 250 identified hazardous substances are carcinogenic. There is no benefit to doing so—don't!

Dextrose, fructose, fruit juice concentrates, glucose, honey, lactose, maltose, molasses, sucrose, sugar (both white and brown), and syrup are examples of sugars (both corn and maple). These should be avoided or taken in moderation. If you must indulge, pair it with protein, fat, or fibre. Simple sugars are digested more healthfully in your body and generate less insulin when consumed in this manner. The best thing to do is to limit your intake of these sugars as much as possible. Although several of my recipes call for a small quantity of brown sugar, I use natural/raw brown sugar, which is only marginally better than brown sugar. Natural brown sugar is made from the initial crystallization of sugarcane and therefore undergoes minimal processing. Regular brown sugar is just refined white sugar with molasses added to it. Moderation is essential. High-fructose corn syrup should be avoided at all costs.

Supplements have not yet been shown to aid in the battle against cancer. On this subject, the jury is still out since not enough data has been collected. Some high-dose supplements may potentially raise the risk of cancer. This is a personal decision that should be taken after doing research and consulting with your doctor. Food is still the greatest source of vitamins and minerals.

Tanning beds have been linked to cancer in humans. So run in the other direction—do not stroll! Use them at your own risk!

Antioxidants may be found in all kinds of tea. White and green teas are less processed than black tea and have higher antioxidant levels. There is conflicting evidence that tea can help prevent cancer. Tea has been shown in labs to combat cancer, but the outcomes in human trials have been mixed. When I was diagnosed, I gave up coffee and switched to green tea. It is common for studies to be mixed. I'd rather err on the side of caution.

Be on the safe side. If it hasn't been shown to hurt me, it may benefit me.

Vegetables are delicious, but their preparation may be perplexing. Brassica vegetables, including broccoli, Brussels sprouts, cauliflower, and green cabbage, have been proven in labs to help prevent cancer. However, recent research has shown that boiling significantly depletes these veggies' cancer-fighting qualities. Steaming, stir-frying, or microwaving them is a superior method to prepare them.

Green beans, beets, and garlic were shown to maintain their antioxidant levels after most cooking techniques in tests. Still, artichokes were the only vegetable that kept their high antioxidant level across all cooking procedures.

Vitamin D may be beneficial in the treatment of some malignancies. Vitamin D is acquired via skin contact with sunlight, supplements, and diet. Still, few foods contain Vitamin D. Vitamin D is found in salmon, sardines, mackerel, cod liver oil, and fortified foods such as milk and cereals. The Vitamin D debate should be addressed with your doctor since recommended Vitamin D levels differ depending on gender and age.

Many physicians now feel that the currently suggested doses are inadequate and advocate for higher levels. Sun exposure is one of the greatest methods to acquire Vitamin D. Still, many variables, including dark skin, age (older individuals have reduced conversion in their skin to create Vitamin D), genetics, obesity, and some medicines, reduce the body's capacity to make Vitamin D. Increased sun exposure raises the risk of skin cancer. At the same time, sunscreen prevents Vitamin D production in the skin. It's all a little perplexing, and who knows for sure? There does not seem to be a definitive solution here. As a result, some personal investigation and a conversation with your doctor are recommended.

FOODS TO TRY

These are items that I aim to include in my regular diet but always consult with your doctor or a professional dietitian first to ensure they are appropriate for you and any special nutritional needs you may have. For example, there is debate about eating soy if you have a history of breast or other hormone-related cancer, the debate over the advantages vs dangers of drinking red wine, and debate over the impact of certain fats (omega-3s) on specific malignancies.

So, in addition to consulting with your physician, I would recommend that you do some extra study on your own for your daily diet. These are foods that have been proven in scientific studies to help fight cancer, and I aim to consume them regularly.

Berries are rich in antioxidants and a good source of many compounds that seem to help prevent cancer.

Citrus fruits include limonoids, which are chemicals found in peels. Under laboratory circumstances, preliminary studies showed that limonoids might prevent and stop cancer.

The molecule Indole-3-Carbinol, or I3C for short, is found in cruciferous vegetables such as cabbage, broccoli, kale, chard, cauliflower, Brussels sprouts, and collard greens. According to research, I3C promotes a process known as apoptosis, which includes the removal of damaged cells from your body. Researchers have also shown I3C to aid in the prevention of cancer cell growth.

Dark chocolate has a lot of antioxidants. It must be dark chocolate, not milk chocolate, and contain at least 70% cacao. If the packaging claims dark chocolate but does not specify the cacao content, it is most likely not at least 70% cacao. Before you get too excited about consuming this meal, keep in mind that moderation is the key. While dark chocolate is beneficial to your health, it is also rich in fat and calories. It is not advised to drink more than 1½ ounces each day.

Garlic, according to research, protects against stomach cancer and lowers the risk of getting colon cancer. However, when garlic is chopped and then cooked quickly, it loses its potential anti-cancer effects. Therefore, always start by preparing the garlic. Then, allow the sliced garlic to rest for at least ten minutes before cooking if it will be crushed, minced, or chopped in a dish. According to studies, allowing garlic to sit, even for a short period, enables it to maintain the majority of its nutritional content.

Green and white teas include two compounds: epigallocatechin gallate (EGCG) and epigallocatechin gallate (EGCC) (EGC). These have been proven in labs to help prevent cancer.

Herbs and spices are often high in antioxidants. For example, one tablespoon of oregano has the same amount of antioxidants as a medium-sized apple. In addition, recent research has shown that oregano has significantly more antioxidants than garlic, which has long been recognized for its antioxidant qualities.

• The most antioxidant-rich fresh herbs include oregano, sage, peppermint, thyme, lemon balm, and marjoram.

• Cloves, allspice, cinnamon, rosemary, thyme, marjoram, saffron, oregano, tarragon, and basil are the dried herbs with the highest antioxidant activity.

Omega-3 fatty acids are classified as EFAs (essential fatty acids). EFAs are essential for human health but cannot be produced by the body. As a result, they must be acquired via diet. Fish and some plant oils contain omega-3 fatty acids. Omega-3s may be found in walnuts, salmon, soybeans, halibut, shrimp, tofu, winter squash, snapper, scallops, and supplements. As I do, if you take supplements, be sure they meet the International Fish Oil Standards Program.

Onions are high in antioxidants, and the stronger the onion, the more antioxidants it contains. Most flavonoids are found in shallots and Western Yellow (an antioxidant found in onions). Furthermore, research has revealed that shallots, Northern Red, Western Yellow, and New York Bold onions have the best potential to prevent cancer development.

Red wine has a high concentration of physiologically active phytochemicals, especially anthocyanins.

Polyphenols are chemicals that are thought to have anti-cancer effects. However, moderation is essential. I no longer drink a 3-4 ounce glass of wine with my supper. Excessive alcohol use has been related to a variety of cancers, according to research. Nonetheless, consuming red wine in moderation has substantial health advantages.

Soy meals are high in phytochemicals, and one kind of phytochemicals, isoflavones, has been shown to help fight cancer in several ways. Isoflavones can only be found in soybeans and soy products, including tofu, soy milk, tempeh, and textured soy protein.

Turmeric is a spice that is widely used in India. According to research, it has anti-cancer characteristics and the potential to prevent cancer development and metastatic illness. If I don't cook with this spice on a particular day, I put it in a gel cap and take it as a supplement.

In general, fruits and vegetables are all healthy and should be included in your diet. Although the items on the list above have been proven to help prevent cancer, all veggies are healthy for you and should be included in your diet. Mix them and enjoy! Remember that phytochemicals are substances found exclusively in plants, and research indicates that the more phytochemicals you consume, the lower your risk of cancer.

AVOIDED FOODS

In research, red meat (beef, lamb, and pig) has been found to cause colon cancer, prostate cancer, breast cancer, and lymphoma. Furthermore, meat that has been chargrilled, blackened, or overcooked at high temperatures is likely to contain carcinogens (agents that cause cancer).

Processed meat: According to the American Institute for Cancer Research and the World Cancer Research Fund's Second Expert Report, processed meat is likely to cause many types of colon cancer. Carcinogens are produced when meat is preserved by smoking, curing, salting, and adding chemical preservatives. Hot dogs, ham, bacon, salami, sausages, and lunch meats are processed meats.

Sugar: Some individuals believe that sugar feeds cancer. That is not correct. Excessive consumption of nonnutritive sugar and refined, simple carbs may increase insulin-like growth (IGF), stimulating cells to expand. IGF is a natural and essential component of the human body. However, too much IGF is harmful.

First and foremost, restrict your sugar intake—no soft drinks, no bakery goods, and no junk food. Try to avoid processed meals at all costs. Refined sugars should be avoided. Avoid simple carbs that rapidly convert to sugar in your body, such as white bread, cookies, sweets, and jams. Second, eat more complex carbs, such as whole grains, fruits, vegetables, beans, and legumes.

Fats may be a bit of a tricky subject. A high-saturated-fat diet has been linked to the development of many illnesses, including cancer. On the other hand, a diet rich in unsaturated fat and low saturated fat has been proven to protect against various illnesses, including cancer. This is another way of saying, eat veggies instead of meat!

Fats are necessary for our bodies, and omega-3s are mentioned in the Foods To Enjoy section. However, a low-fat diet is associated with cancer prevention. Therefore, try to limit your fat consumption to no more than 20% of your entire daily food intake.

Dairy products (other than skim or nonfat), margarine, lard, animal fats (excluding fish), and vegetable oils are all fats to avoid (except olive and canola oils). That means avoiding most baked products and snacks unless they are prepared healthily.

Omega-6s are likewise classified as EFAs (essential fatty acids); however, consuming them requires a delicate balance since certain omega-6s are harmful if eaten in excess. This is especially true for linoleic acid, which is present in a variety of vegetable oils. Because we consume so much junk food in the United States, our diets are too rich in omega-6 fats. A balanced diet that includes various foods high in omega-3 and omega-6 fats is essential for optimum health. However, the ratio should be close to 3:1 omega-6s to omega-3s. In the United States, the ratios may be as high as 50:1! Is it any surprise that we are in the grip of a cancer epidemic? Avoid pro-inflammatory, refined, and hydrogenated omega-6s found in maize, soy, sunflower, and safflower oils, as well as margarine. You can obtain omega-6s from olive oil, almonds, soybeans, and walnuts, but remember that balance is key when it comes to omega-6s.

Salt: According to the American Institute for Cancer Research and The World Cancer Research Fund's Second Expert Report, salt has been shown to cause stomach and liver cancer, particularly via the consumption of salt-preserved, salted, or salty foods. Their advice is to consume fewer than 2 grams of salt per day from all sources. Read food labels and limit your salt intake to no more than 2,000 milligrams (2 grams) each day. This amounts to a little less than one teaspoon of salt. Furthermore, individuals 51 years of age or older, African Americans, and those with high blood pressure, diabetes, or chronic renal disease should not consume more than 1500 mg per day, according to the USDA.

I think that surgery and chemotherapy healed my cancer, but altering my diet has prevented it from returning.

BREAKFAST

French Toast with Stuffing

You'll note that this part is very short. That's because, like most people, I had the same breakfast every day. I typically eat a bowl of whole-grain cereal with banana, berries, and soy milk. I do this for two reasons: the time limitations of getting ready for work on a weekday morning, and whole-grain cereal and fruit are healthier options. On weekends, when I have more time, I like to have more variety and fun with my breakfasts. But, again, I only do this in moderation.

The issue with most traditional breakfasts is that they are high in unhealthy fats, processed meats, and sweets. But, we can still have delicious breakfasts, don't worry! This section's dishes are healthier adaptations of old favourites.

Florentine English Muffins with Egg Whites

This may fulfil your desire for Eggs Benedict without jeopardizing your health. On the contrary, these open-faced sandwiches stuffed with spinach are a pleasant Sunday morning treat!

- 2 English muffins (whole wheat)
- 1/4 cup grated cheese (part-skim mozzarella, veggie, or soy)
- 2 tbsp canola oil
- 4 cups loosely packed, chopped fresh spinach
- 8 large egg whites
- 1 tbsp. chopped pimento
- 1 teaspoon cornstarch

- 34 cup fat-free milk
- 1 teaspoon fresh lemon juice
- 1 tablespoon fresh chopped
- parsley, flat-leaf
- seasoned with salt & pepper
- Spray with canola oil

Preheat the oven to 250°F. Toast the muffins gently after splitting them. Place the pieces on a cookie sheet side by side. Spread the cheese evenly over the muffins and place in the oven to melt.

Sauté spinach in 1 tablespoon canola oil in a medium pan over medium-high heat until it wilts. Set aside and season with salt and pepper to taste.

Place another medium skillet over low heat and coat with canola oil spray. Mix in the egg whites. Over the eggs, scatter the chopped pimento. Cover the pan with a lid until the eggs are done (to allow the eggs to get fluffy). Remove the lid, turn off the heat, and put it aside.

Serve the muffins with the sautéed spinach on top. On top of the spinach, place the eggs. Return the cookie sheet to the oven to stay warm.

Whisk together the cornstarch and 1 tablespoon canola oil in a small pan until the cornstarch dissolves. Heat a skillet over high heat. Add the milk gently, whisking continuously until the liquid starts to boil and thicken. Reduce the heat to low and continue cooking for 1 minute, whisking continuously. Take the pan off the heat. Incorporate the lemon juice and parsley—season with salt and pepper to taste.

Remove the muffins from the oven and arrange them on serving plates. Distribute the white sauce evenly over the muffins. On the side, serve with fresh, seasonal fruit.

If the white sauce becomes too thick, whisk in a bit more milk. If not served immediately, the sauce will thicken.

Serves 4

Florentine eggs

This dish fulfils my desire for a whole egg on occasion. It tastes rich and delicious while being low in fat. Previously, I would have had two eggs for the morning. Now I'm ok with one...and only on rare occasions.

- 2 tbsp canola oil
- 2 tbsp. coarsely chopped onion
- 4 cups loosely packed, chopped fresh spinach
- 2 tbsp. cheese, shredded (part-skim mozzarella, veggie, or soy)
- 1 teaspoon cornstarch
- 34 cup fat-free milk
- 1 teaspoon grated low-fat
- The parmesan cheese
- 1 tablespoon fresh chopped
- parsley, flat-leaf
- seasoned with salt & pepper
- Spray with canola oil
- two eggs

- seasoned with salt & pepper

1. Preheat the oven to 250°F. In a medium-sized pan, sauté onions in 1 tablespoon canola oil over medium-high heat. Cook, occasionally stirring until the onions are tender. Add the spinach and simmer until it wilts—season with salt and pepper to taste. Divide the spinach mixture evenly between two oven-safe au gratin dishes (or onto 2 oven-safe plates). Place each spinach mixture in a preheated oven and top with 1 tablespoon shredded cheese.

2. Whisk together the cornstarch and 1 tablespoon canola oil in a small pan until the cornstarch dissolves. Heat a skillet over high heat. Add the milk gently, whisking continuously until the liquid starts to boil and thicken. Reduce the heat to low and continue cooking for 1 minute, whisking continuously. Take the pan off the heat. Incorporate the Parmesan cheese and parsley. Season with salt and pepper to taste. Place aside.

3. They are using a canola oil spray, coat a nonstick skillet. Place a pan over very low heat and crack 2 eggs into it, taking care not to break the yolks. Cook, covered until the eggs are done, but the yolks are still tender. Remove the lid from the eggs and turn off the heat in the skillet.

4. Remove the spinach from the oven with care. On each dish, place 1 egg on top of the spinach. Distribute the sauce evenly over each egg. Serve right away.

Serves 2

Burrito for Breakfast

This burrito is quick and simple to make, and it can even be eaten on the move if you leave off the sauce at the end.

- 1 medium diced onion
- ½ medium diced green pepper

- 1½ medium diced red pepper
- 1 diced tomato
- 2 whole eggs + 8 egg whites (whisked)
- 4 whole wheat flour tortillas, 10 in.
- 4 oz. shredded cheese (part-skim mozzarella, veggie, or soy)
- seasoned with salt & pepper
- ¼ teaspoon coarsely chopped spicy chilli pepper (optional)
- Spray with canola oil
- ½ cup salsa
- 1 peeled and sliced avocado
- ½ cup nonfat plain yoghurt

Preheat the oven to 300°F. Canola oil coat a medium skillet generously. Sauté the onion, peppers, and tomato in the sprayed skillet until the onions are transparent and the peppers are tender (about 5 minutes). Cook until the eggs are done. If desired, season with spicy chilli pepper. Season with salt and pepper to taste. Warm the tortillas in the microwave or on the stovetop. Fill a heated tortilla with the egg mixture and cheese. Form a burrito by rolling up the tortilla. To melt the cheese, place the burritos in a preheated oven for 3 minutes. Remove from the oven and serve with salsa and avocado on top. On the side, serve nonfat yoghurt.

Serves 4

Omelet Veggie Egg White

Covering the omelette traps steam and keeps it fluffy. You won't miss the yolk at all!

- 1 small onion, coarsely chopped
- ½ red pepper, coarsely chopped
- 1 cup sliced mushrooms
- 1 medium tomato, coarsely chopped
- ½ finely chopped green pepper
- 5 egg whites + 1 whole egg
- 2 tbsp flat-leaf parsley, chopped
- 1 tbsp. grated Parmesan cheese (low-fat)
- seasoned with salt & pepper
- Spray with canola oil
- ¼ cup salsa (optional)

1. Heat a medium skillet over medium heat, sprayed with canola oil spray. Cook until the onions, peppers, and mushrooms are tender (about 5 minutes). Season with salt and pepper to taste. Cook for another 2 minutes before removing from the heat. Whisk the egg whites and egg until foamy in a medium bowl, then pour into a medium skillet coated with canola oil spray. Heat the skillet over low heat. Cover with a tight-fitting lid. When the eggs have started to cook but are still soft, add the cooked veggies and sprinkle with parsley and Parmesan.
2. Replace the lid and simmer until the eggs are done. Fold the omelette using a spatula. If preferred, cut in half and serve with salsa.

Serves 2

Pizza for Breakfast

This is a great breakfast or dinner, for that matter!

- One ½-inch rolled out
- Pizza Dough Made From Whole Wheat
- Dusting with cornmeal
- 1 tbsp of canola oil
- ½ medium chopped red onion
- ½ cup sliced fresh mushrooms
- 2 cups chopped fresh spinach
- 1 pre-cooked baked potato, chopped into 12-inch pieces
- 6 egg whites
- 2 tablespoons finely chopped
- parsley, flat-leaf
- a quarter-cup of shredded cheese (part-skim mozzarella, veggie, or soy)
- Spray with canola oil
- Seasoned with salt & pepper
- ½ cup salsa (optional)
- Flakes of hot pepper (optional)

1. Preheat the oven to 400°F. Sprinkle some cornmeal on a pizza paddle. Roll out the pizza dough and place it on the paddle. If you don't have a pizza paddle, put the pizza dough on a cooling rack as least as big as the flattened out dough.
2. Slide the dough straight onto the oven rack in the middle of

the oven using the paddle. If you're using a cooling rack, put it in the middle of the oven. Cook for 3 minutes or until the dough is somewhat firm. Once the toppings are on the pizza, you may simply take it off the paddle or cooling rack. Remove the dough from the oven when it is somewhat hard. Do not switch off the oven.

3. In a medium pan, caramelize the onion in the canola oil (about 20 minutes, onions should be soft and slightly brown). Combine the mushrooms, spinach, and potato in a mixing bowl. Cook until the spinach has wilted and the potatoes have developed some colour. Continue to cook, constantly stirring, until the egg whites are scrambled. Season with salt and pepper to taste.

4. Spread the egg mixture evenly over the pizza dough, leaving a 1/2-inch border on both sides. Garnish with chopped parsley and cheese if desired. Return to the oven and bake for 7-10 minutes, or until the crust is crisp and the cheese has melted. Remove from the oven, slice, and serve! If desired, top with salsa and hot pepper flakes.

Serves 2

Pancakes with Cornmeal

For breakfast, I nearly always have cereal with berries and soy milk. On weekends, I sometimes like pancakes as a treat. Here's a healthier alternative that I can enjoy without feeling guilty.

- 1 cup cornmeal (yellow)
- ½ CUP WHOLE WHOLE WHEAT FLOUR
- ½ cup quick oats
- 1 tbsp. raw brown sugar
- 1 tbsp baking powder

- 1 teaspoon sea salt
- 2 egg whites
- 1 cup nonfat plain yoghurt
- ½ cup fat-free milk
- Spray with canola oil

1. Preheat a grill or big skillet over medium heat. When a few droplets of water dance on the grill or pan, it is ready.
2. Mix the dry ingredients well. Mix in the egg whites, yoghurt, and milk until well mixed. Add just the quantity of milk you need to make the batter you want. Thinner batter results in thinner pancakes, whereas thicker batter results in thicker pancakes.

Serves 4

Canola oil sprays a hot grill or pan. Spoon 2 teaspoons batter into skillet for each pancake, working in batches. Cook until golden brown on both sides, approximately 2 minutes on each side. Because there is no oil in these pancakes, you will need to re-spray the grill with canola oil after each batch. Serve with a compote of fresh fruit.

Serves 4

Compote de fruits frais

This is a great healthy substitute for syrup on pancakes or French toast. It's high in antioxidants, warm, welcoming, and delicious!

- 1 cup blueberries, fresh
- 1 cup sliced fresh strawberries
- 1 sliced banana

- 1 diced peach
- 1 teaspoon ground cinnamon
- ½ lemon juice
- Spray with canola oil

1. Spray a medium skillet with canola oil spray and add all of the ingredients. Cook over low heat until the sauce thickens and all of the ingredients have melded together. Serve with cornmeal pancakes, oatcakes, or stuffed french toast.

Serves 4

Green Omelette

This omelette has so much cancer-fighting broccoli and spinach that I should have named it the antioxidant omelette! This not only makes a lovely appearance when topped with salsa, but it also tastes delicious.

- 1 tbsp of canola oil
- 1 cup broccoli, finely chopped
- 1 handful chopped scallions
- 2 whole eggs + 5 egg whites
- ¼ cup fat-free milk
- 1 cup chopped spinach
- ¼ cup chopped flat-leaf parsley
- Spray with canola oil
- ½ cup salsa to serve as a garnish (optional)

Allow canola oil to heat up in a small pan over medium heat. In a pan, sauté the broccoli and scallions for 4-5 minutes, or until the scallions begin to turn translucent. Then, take the pan off the heat.

Combine the egg whites, eggs, and milk in a mixing bowl. Heat a medium skillet over low heat, sprayed with canola oil spray. Pour in the eggs. Layer veggies on one side of the pan after approximately 1 minute, when the eggs begin to cook. Continue to cook on low heat with a tight-fitting lid. This allows the eggs to inflate up. When

When the omelette is completely cooked, turn the side without the filling over onto the side with the filling. Take the pan off the heat. Serve with salsa or sliced tomatoes on the side.

Serves 2

Scrambled Eggs with Indian Spices

Here's a different take on the classic egg scramble. Turmeric, which is now being studied in several studies, is thought by some researchers to prevent and delay developing various cancers.

- 1 medium unpeeled unpeeled unpeeled unpeeled unpeeled unpeeled unpeeled un
- 1 medium coarsely diced onion
- 1 cup chopped fresh spinach
- 2 medium diced tomatoes
- 6 egg whites
- ½ teaspoon curry powder
- ½ teaspoon of turmeric
- ¾ teaspoon cumin
- 1 tablespoon chopped cilantro

- Spray with canola oil

Spray a medium pan well with canola oil spray before adding the potato and onion. Cook until the potatoes are golden and the onions are transparent (about 10 minutes). Stir in the spinach and tomatoes until the spinach wilts. In a medium mixing bowl, combine the egg whites, curry, turmeric, and cumin. Mix thoroughly in the skillet. Cook until the eggs are completely cooked over low heat. Garnish with fresh cilantro. Serve hot.

Serves 2

Casserole with Hash Browns and Eggs

I don't eat eggs very frequently, but this is a semi-healthy variation of a fattier original. Egg casseroles are often high in fat due to the addition of cheese and sausages. Therefore, I mostly utilize egg whites and low-fat cheese. This is not a weekend meal, but it is a wonderful dish to serve with guests since it can be made the day before, wrapped in plastic wrap, and baked the following morning. Before they depart, my visitors always ask for the recipe!

- 2 tbsp canola oil
- 1 big sliced onion
- 1 chopped green pepper
- 1 chopped red pepper
- 2 cups shredded white potatoes, unpeeled
- 2 cups peeled and shredded sweet potatoes
- ½ egg whites + 4 eggs

- 1-quart non-fat milk
- ¼ cup flat-leaf parsley, chopped
- 1 cup grated cheese (part-skim mozzarella, veggie, or soy)
- ¼ cup low-fat grated Parmesan
- Spray with canola oil
- Seasoned with salt & pepper

2. Preheat the oven to 350°F. Using a paper towel, pat the shredded potatoes dry.

3. In a large pan, heat the canola oil and add the onion, green pepper, and red pepper. Cook until the veggies are tender. Place aside.

4. Coat a big pan or skillet with canola oil spray. Mix in both kinds of shredded potatoes. While the potatoes are cooking, season them with salt and pepper. Cook for 10 minutes over medium heat, then flip the potatoes and cook for another 10 minutes. Set aside when they are soft.

5. Combine the whole eggs, egg whites, and milk in a mixing bowl. Add the parsley and mix well.

6. Using a canola oil spray, coat a 9 x 13 baking dish. Cover the bottom of the skillet with hash browns. Over the potatoes, layer the sautéed onion and peppers. Top the veggies with the crumbled cheese. Pour the egg mixture over the top of the casserole, covering it completely. Sprinkle with Parmesan cheese on top.

7. Cook for 45 minutes in a preheated oven, covered with aluminium foil. Remove the foil and continue to simmer for another 15 minutes, or until the potatoes are tender. Serve right away.

Serves 6-8

Pancakes with Oatmeal

Because they are prepared without the usual fats and sweets, these pancakes are guilt-free. After a couple of them, you may not want the regular type anymore!

- ½ cup soy or nonfat milk
- ½ teaspoon of vinegar
- 1 cup whole wheat white flour
- 1 cup oats, old-fashioned
- 1 tbsp. raw brown sugar
- 1 tsp. baking soda
- ¼ tsp of salt
- 2 big, gently beaten egg whites
- 1 cup nonfat plain yoghurt
- Spray with canola oil

Preheat a grill or a big skillet over medium-high heat. When a few droplets of water placed on the surface dance, it's ready. Pour the vinegar into the milk to create a buttermilk substitute. Place aside.

Combine the flour, oatmeal, sugar, baking soda, and salt in a large mixing basin. In a separate small dish, mix the egg whites, fake buttermilk, and yoghurt. Pour the wet ingredients into the dry ingredients and well combine.

Canola oil sprays the hot griddle or skillet. Working in batches to prevent the oil from burning, pour 2 teaspoons batter onto a griddle or skillet for each pancake. Cook until golden brown on both sides, approximately 2 minutes on each side. Because there is no oil in these pancakes, you will need to re-spray the griddle or skillet with canola oil after each batch. Serve with a compote of fresh fruit.

Serves 3-4

Hot Cereal with Whole Grain

Make a week's worth of breakfast in advance and keep it in the refrigerator to save time in the morning.

4 cups water

- ½ cup cracked whole grain wheat
- ½ cup rolled oats
- 1 teaspoon ground cinnamon
- ¼ cup raisin

Bring the water to a boil in a big saucepan. Combine the oats, wheat, and cinnamon in a mixing bowl. Reduce the heat to a gentle simmer and cover. Continue to cook for 20-30 minutes, or until the water has been absorbed and the grain has reached the appropriate consistency. Stir in the raisins well. Remove from the heat and serve right away, or cool and keep in an airtight jar in the refrigerator. Before serving, reheat the dish.

When reheating, add a little water to thin it out.

Serves 6-8

Pancakes with Ricotta and Blueberries

This is a lovely, unique Sunday morning meal that is ideal for serving visitors. The blueberries are hot and juicy, and the pancakes are light and fluffy. In addition to making these pancakes a delicious treat, blueberries have been shown in recent research to help suppress cancer cells.

- 1 cup soy or nonfat milk
- 1 lemon juice

- ¼ cup whole wheat white flour
- ¼ cup quick oats
- 1 tsp brown sugar, raw
- 1 tsp. baking powder
- ½ tsp baking soda
- ½ teaspoon ground nutmeg
- ½ teaspoon of salt
- ¾ cup ricotta cheese, nonfat or part-skim
- 1 lemon's zest
- ¼ cc orange juice
- 2 egg whites, big
- ½ teaspoon vanilla extract
- ¾ cup blueberries, fresh or frozen (unthawed)
- Spray with canola oil

Preheat the oven to 250°F. Make fake buttermilk by squeezing lemon into milk. Place aside.

Preheat a grill or big skillet over medium-high heat. When you put a few water droplets over the grill or pan, the water dances.

In a large mixing bowl, combine the dry ingredients (flour, oatmeal, sugar, baking powder, baking soda, salt, and nutmeg). Next, in a separate dish, whisk together the ricotta, fake buttermilk, lemon zest, orange juice, egg whites, and vanilla extract. Whisk until well mixed and foamy. Next, combine the dry and wet ingredients in a mixing bowl. Blueberries should be folded in at this point.

Spray the griddle or skillet with canola oil spray once it's heated. Spoon 1/4 cup batter onto the griddle for each pancake immediately, so the oil does not burn. Cook the pancake until the bottom is golden brown and bubbles form on the top. When bubbles appear, turn the pancakes and cook for another 2-3 minutes on the other side. Repeat with each fresh batch, spraying the skillet with canola oil spray until all batters have been utilized.

While the next batch cooks, place the cooked pancakes immediately on the oven rack. These pancakes are naturally wet, and the additional cooking time in the oven at a moderate temperature dries them out to the ideal consistency. Serve immediately with Fresh Fruit Compote.

18 pancakes are produced.

French Toast with Stuffing

This is a rich, delicious dessert that is very simple to prepare. Years ago, in Wichita, Kansas, I used to go to a tiny restaurant that offered a premium peanut butter and jelly sandwich with bananas and almonds. This is my lighter version. The fruit within the bread becomes warm and mushy, and there are many healthy things inside. Blueberries, walnuts, cinnamon, and almond butter are high antioxidants, which can protect against cancer.

- 4 whole-grain or whole wheat bread slices
- 4 tbsp almond butter
- 2 bananas, thinly sliced longways
- 4 big strawberries, thinly sliced
- ½ cup blueberries, fresh
- 2 eggs
- 1 cup soy or nonfat milk

- 1 teaspoon ground cinnamon
- ½ teaspoon of salt
- ½ tsp almond extract
- 1 big orange's zest
- 1 big lemon's zest
- ¼ cup toasted chopped walnuts
- a sprinkling of powdered sugar (optional)
- Spray with canola oil

Spread almond butter equally over four slices of bread to help keep the French toast together. Next, place the sliced bananas on top of the almond butter on two slices of bread. Next, place sliced strawberries on top of banana slices, then blueberries on top of the strawberries.

Make two sandwiches by layering the almond butter-covered bread on top of the fruit-layered bread. Lightly press the sandwiches together, so they stay together when dipped in the egg mixture. Cut the sandwich diagonally into quarters.

Whisk together the egg, milk, cinnamon, salt, and almond extract in a medium mixing dish. Coat the sandwich quarters completely in the egg mixture.

Preheat a grill or skillet to medium-high heat. Spray the prepared skillet or pan with canola oil spray when you're ready to put the French toast on it. Place the dipped sandwich quarters on a grill or pan and fry for 3 minutes on each side, turning once, until golden brown on both sides.

When done, sprinkle with zests and toasted walnuts. If preferred, sprinkle with a thin sprinkling of powdered sugar. Serve with a compote of fresh fruit.

Serves 2-3

SNACKS AND SMOOTHIES

Smoothie with Pineapple, Banana, and Cacao

Unfortunately, snacks are often our modern-day nutritional disaster. We have a penchant for foods that are sweet, salty, and high in refined and hydrogenated omega-6 fatty acids (Foods to Avoid). It's time to alter that, to retrain our palates to appreciate healthier versions of our favourite snacks in between meals.

Most of the time, I nibble on raw nuts such as almonds or walnuts or home-popped popcorn made without butter or harmful oils. When I want something different, I resort to my new favourites, such as smoothies, frozen fruits, and roasted garbanzo beans.

Smoothies are very simple to prepare. Simply combine the ingredients in a blender, add ice, and mix until smooth and icy. Unfortunately, many smoothies, particularly those purchased at coffee shops, contain hidden fat and sugars. Although shop signage may state that they are healthful, this is not always the case.

These are a handful of my favourite smoothie recipes, although smoothies can be a versatile meal. Whatever fruit or drink you have in your refrigerator will most likely create a delicious snack. Consider these recipes to be a starting point. Begin with my suggestions, and then use your creativity to create some liquid magic!

Smoothie with Almond Butter

Almond butter is a nutritional powerhouse since it is composed entirely of almonds. Almonds have a low saturated fat content (the bad stuff), a high monounsaturated fat content (the healthy stuff), and no transfat (the worst stuff). This smoothie has the flavour of a thick, luscious shake.

- 1 cup nonfat plain yoghurt

- 1 cup milk (nonfat, soy, or almond)
- 1 banana, peeled, sliced, and frozen
- 2 tbsp almond butter
- 1 teaspoon maple syrup
- ½ teaspoon ground cinnamon
- 1 cup cubes ice
- Blend all of the ingredients in a blender until smooth.
- **Serves 2**

Smoothie with apricots and pineapples

Apricots are high in vitamins A and C, as well as beta-carotene. So the apricot is a little fruit with a huge nutritional punch.

- ½ cup canned unsweetened crushed pineapple
- 3 pitted fresh apricots or 3 dried apricots
- 2 big strawberries, cut off the tips
- ½ bananas, peeled, quartered, and frozen
- 1 cup nonfat plain yoghurt
- 1 cup cubes ice

Blend all of the ingredients in a blender until smooth.

Serves 2

Smoothie with Mango

Mangoes are rich in phytochemicals, fibre, vitamins and are low in fat. Mangoes also contain beta-carotene, which has been proven in studies to help decrease the incidence of some malignancies. If you drink one of these, you'll feel as if you're on a tropical vacation!

- 1 big orange, peeled and seeded
- 1 peeled, sliced and frozen fresh mango
- 1 peeled, cut in thirds, and frozen banana
- 1 cup nonfat plain yoghurt
- 1 cup nonfat or soy milk ¾ -1 cup

For this smoothie, you'll need to freeze the mango and banana ahead of time. Then, instead of using ice, the frozen fruit will thicken the smoothie.

Blend all of the ingredients in a blender until smooth. Add the quantity of milk required to get the desired consistency.

Serves 2

Smoothie with Bananas and Oranges

Bananas are often referred to as the "ideal fruit," and they are undoubtedly one of the most popular. They include many fibres, potassium, and vitamin C. Oranges are also abundant in Vitamin C, calcium, beta-carotene, and other minerals. This is a basic, old-fashioned banana smoothie recipe that will satisfy on a hot summer day. However, sometimes keeping things simple is preferable.

- 1 banana, peeled and divided into thirds
- 1 big (or 2 small) orange, peeled, seeded, and quartered
- ¼ cc orange juice
- 1 cup nonfat plain yoghurt

- 1 cup cubes ice

Blend all of the ingredients in a blender until smooth.

Serves 2

Smoothie with Berries

Berries are often regarded as a superfood by many. According to research, berries have one of the greatest antioxidant levels of any food and include phytochemicals that help prevent cancer.

- 1 cup freshly squeezed orange juice
- 1 cup nonfat plain yoghurt
- 1 cup strawberries, fresh
- 1 cup blueberries, fresh
- ½ cup ripe raspberries
- 1 cup cubes ice

Blend all of the ingredients in a blender until smooth.

Serves 2

Smoothie with Pineapple, Banana, and Cacao

This is a delicious, thick smoothie that tastes like a chocolate shake. Simply place any overripe bananas in the freezer and store them for when you want to create this smoothie. Next, I open a can of pineapple, divide it into two plastic freezer bags, and freeze them until they're ready to use.

- 1 frozen ripe banana

- ¾ cup unsweetened frozen pineapple chunks (fresh, canned, or packaged)

- 1 cup nonfat plain yoghurt

- 1 cup soy or nonfat milk

- 1 tbsp cacao powder, unsweetened

- 1 teaspoon maple syrup

- 1 tsp vanilla extract

- 4 cubes of ice

Blend all of the ingredients in a blender until smooth.

Serves 2

Smoothie with Kale

Kale may seem odd in a smoothie, but it really works well when combined with frozen fruit. Kale has been proven to help strengthen your immune system and lower your chances of developing several malignancies. In addition, it's a fun way to consume cruciferous veggies!

- 1 peeled, cut in thirds, and frozen banana

- 10 kale leaves, with a big vein through the centre removed

- 1 peeled, diced, and frozen mango

- 1 cup peeled, diced, and frozen pineapple

- 1 cup cubes ice

- 1 cup freshly squeezed orange juice

- 1 cup pineapple puree
- Blend all of the ingredients in a blender until smooth.

Serves 2

Garbanzo Beans, Roasted

Garbanzo beans (chickpeas) are rich in fibre and protein and shown in tests to prevent some malignancies. In addition, these little beans are packed with minerals. These beans are delicious as a snack on their own or over a fresh salad.

- 2 cans (15 oz.) garbanzo beans (chickpeas)
- 2 tablespoons cumin
- 2 tsp. granulated garlic
- 1 tablespoon chilli powder
- 4 tsp olive oil
- Spray with canola oil
- Seasoned with salt & pepper

Preheat the oven to 375°F. Garbanzo beans should be drained and rinsed well with cold water. Dry the beans with a paper towel until no water remains and the beans are completely dry.

Toss garbanzo beans with olive oil and spices in a medium-sized mixing basin. I am using a canola oil spray, coat a baking sheet. Arrange on a baking sheet in a single layer. Bake for 45 minutes, stirring periodically until they are slightly browned and crisp.

If desired, season with salt and pepper.

Serves 3-4

Smoothie with peaches

Because of their pits, peaches are known as stone fruits. Stone fruits are high in phenols (organic chemicals), encouraging laboratory studies against breast cancer cells.

- 2 pitted, chunked, frozen peaches
- 1 cup nonfat plain yoghurt
- ½ cup freshly squeezed orange juice
- ½ cup soy or nonfat milk
- 1 teaspoon maple syrup
- 1 cup cubes ice

Blend all of the ingredients in a blender until smooth.

Serves 2

Trail Mix is a healthy snack.

Making your trail mix is easy and tastes better than shop purchased. Here, moderation is required. Even though the components are nutritious, almonds and dark chocolate are rich in calories. Maintaining a healthy weight is critical for cancer prevention.

- ½ cup quick-cooking oats
- 1 teaspoon ground cinnamon
- Spray with canola oil
- ½ cup uncooked almonds
- ½cup uncooked walnuts

- ½ cup toasted pecans
- ½ cup raisin
- ½ cup uncooked sunflower seed kernels
- 2 oz. dark chocolate
- Cacao with a cacao content of 70% or above, ¼-inch chunks

Preheat the oven to 350°F. Combine cinnamon and quick oats in a small bowl. To help cinnamon cling to the oats, spritz them with canola oil spray. Combine thoroughly. On a cookie sheet, evenly distribute the oats. On another cookie sheet, equally, distribute the almonds and walnuts. Toast both cookie sheets in a preheated oven for 10-15 minutes. Be cautious not to overheat. Take the pan out of the oven. Allow for 1 minute of cooling.

In a medium mixing dish, combine the oats, almonds, and walnuts. Next, combine the pecans, raisins, and sunflower seed kernels in a mixing bowl. Combine thoroughly. Finally, add the chocolate and thoroughly combine. Because the nuts are still hot from the oven, the chocolate will melt somewhat, forming tiny, delicious clusters. Spread the mixture evenly on one of the cookie sheets and chill until the chocolate sets. When the chocolate has hardened, it may be taken from the refrigerator.

It serves 12 people.

BREAD

CORNBREAD

Irish Soda Bread (Whole Wheat)

Most mass-produced, processed bread nowadays are devoid of nutrition and include needless chemicals and additives. Check out the Nutrition Facts label on a loaf of bread the next time you go shopping. The bread will most likely include high fructose corn syrup, other sweets, and a slew of chemicals. All of this is in your bread and will enter your body. No, thank you!

If you opt to purchase bread instead of baking it, start reading the labels. Many new artisan breads are prepared with few ingredients, including whole grains, and are meant to be bought and consumed immediately away, rather than being processed to sit on a shelf for days.

When time allows, attempt to bake your bread to eliminate unnecessary ingredients and chemicals. Making bread is easy and doesn't need any physical effort. When dealing with yeast dough, there is a waiting time, but the effort itself is little.

This section's bread is prepared using flours other than white and with little or no vegetable oils or butter. Some are snack bread, some are sandwich bread, while others are excellent as a side dish. Please keep in mind that none of these bread, including the coffee cake bread, are very sweet. Sugars are included in my Foods to Avoid section. Therefore I use them sparingly or not at all. As I mentioned in the introduction, the more you avoid sugary sweet foods, the less you will want them.

It is important to note that calories must still be addressed even if the loaves are made with healthy components. According to the American Institute for Cancer Research and The World Cancer Research Fund's Second Expert Report, there is strong evidence that body fat raises the risk of some malignancies. They advise people to keep healthy body weight. There's no need to completely shun bread. Moderation is essential.

For my bread recipes, I use white whole wheat flour. It is made from white spring wheat rather than red wheat. It mimics the texture of conventional all-purpose white flour more closely. However, unlike white flour, it does not have the bran and germ removed; thus, it is still high in nutrients. It should be easy to find in your local grocery these days.

Let us return to bread as the staff of life rather than the shaft of existence.

Muffins with apples, carrots, and raisins

This muffin recipe has no trans fats. Instead, the applesauce and yoghurt provide moisture. Some studies have shown that high-fat diets increase the risk of cancer.

- 2 cups whole wheat white flour
- 1 cup quick oats
- 1 cup bran (oat or wheat)
- 1 tbsp baking powder
- 1 teaspoon cinnamon powder
- 1 teaspoon ground nutmeg
- ½ tsp ground cloves
- 1 teaspoon sea salt
- 1 big grated carrot
- 2 apples, peeled and coarsely diced

- A cup of raisins
- ¼ cup applesauce, unsweetened
- 1 cup nonfat plain yoghurt
- 2 egg whites
- 1 teaspoon vanilla extract
- Spray with canola oil

Preheat the oven to 375°F. Combine the flour, oatmeal, bran, baking soda, spices, and salt in a mixing bowl.

As well as salt Combine carrots, apples, and raisins in a mixing bowl. Stir in the applesauce, yoghurt, egg whites, and vanilla extract until thoroughly combined.

Spray two standard ½-cup muffin tins with canola oil spray, then fill each cup 34 per cent full. Bake for 20 to 23 minutes, or until a knife inserted into the middle comes out clean. Cool for 5 minutes in the pan on a wire rack. Remove the muffins from the oven and set them aside to cool slightly. Serve hot.

24 muffins are produced.

Banana Cinnamon Bread

Cinnamon, the seemingly benign little spice in your kitchen cupboard, may help control your blood sugar, decrease your cholesterol, and (according to new research) prevent the development of leukaemia and lymphoma cancer cells. After all, who can resist the aroma of fresh cinnamon bread baking on a Sunday morning?

- 2 cups whole wheat white flour
- 1 tbsp. raw brown sugar

- ¼ cup whole wheat germ
- ½ teaspoon of salt
- 1 teaspoon baking powder
- ¼ tsp baking soda
- 2 egg whites
- ¼ teaspoon cinnamon
- ½ cup nonfat plain yoghurt
- 1 ripe banana, peeled and mashed
- A quarter cup skim milk
- ¼ cup of canola oil
- 1/3 cup raisin
- 1/3 cup toasted walnuts
- Spray with canola oil
- Preheat the oven to 350°F.

Combine the dry ingredients (flour, sugar, wheat germ, salt, baking powder, baking soda, cinnamon) in a large mixing basin and mix thoroughly.

Whisk together the wet ingredients (egg whites, skim milk, oil, and yoghurt) in a small dish. Whisk in the banana until thoroughly combined.

Combine the wet and dry ingredients in a mixing bowl. Mix in the raisins and walnuts well.

Coat a 9-inch loaf pan with canola oil spray. Fill the loaf pan halfway with batter. Bake for 40-45 minutes, or until the top of the bread is brown, and the loaf sounds hollow when tapped. Allow the bread to cool completely before removing it from the pan.

Makes one loaf

Ciabatta Baguette

- 3 cup whole wheat bread flour
- 1 cup white unbleached flour
- 2 cups water (110-115 degrees F.)
- 1 pound active dry yeast
- 1 teaspoon sea salt
- 1 tbsp natural sugar
- Dusted with flour
- Spray with canola oil

Allow yeast to dissolve in ½ cups of warm water for 10 minutes.

After combining all of the other ingredients (including 1½ cups warm water), add the yeast mixture. Stir the ingredients until it forms a smooth but sticky dough. Form a ball with your hands. Spray a clean surface with canola oil spray and knead the dough ball on it for 5 minutes, or until the dough is smooth. If required, add a little amount of flour while kneading.

Spray a medium-sized mixing basin with canola oil spray, then add the dough. Cover with plastic wrap and set aside for 1 hour, or until the dough has doubled in size.

Empty bowl contents onto a floured, smooth surface. Divide the dough in half and shape it into two 10 inch loaves. Place the loaves on a baking sheet that has been buttered.

There should be at least 4 inches between them. Allow to rise until twice in size, then gently cover plastic wrap (about 1 hour).

Preheat the oven to 450°F. Water should be sprayed on the loaves. 20-25 minutes in the oven

Makes two loaves.

Coffee Cake with Poppy Seeds and Citrus

This mid-morning snack contains nonfat yoghurt, which adds moisture to the cake without adding fat. It's not too sweet, but it's filling and won't leave you hungry an hour later.

- 3 cups whole wheat white flour
- 1 cup quick oats
- 1 teaspoon baking powder
- 1 tsp. baking soda
- ½ cup unrefined brown sugar
- 3 tbsp poppy seeds
- 2 egg whites
- 1 cup soy or nonfat milk
- 1 orange, zipped and juiced
- 1 lemon, zipped and juiced
- 1 lime juice
- 1 cup nonfat plain yoghurt
- 1 teaspoon sea salt

- Spray with canola oil
- Preheat the oven to 375°F.

In a large mixing bowl, combine the flour, oatmeal, baking powder, baking soda, brown sugar, and salt.

Add poppy seeds (leave out 1 tablespoon poppy seeds and 1 tablespoon brown sugar) and thoroughly combine. Mix the egg whites, milk, lemon (zest and juice), orange (zest and juice), lime juice, and a separate dish, yoghurt. Mix the wet and dry components.

Spray a 9" square cake pan with canola oil spray and fill with a coffee cake batter. Sprinkle with the remaining poppy seeds and brown sugar on top and bake in a preheated oven for 45-50 minutes, or until a toothpick inserted into the centre comes out clean.

Serves 16-20

Cornbread

- A cup of cornmeal
- 1 cup whole wheat white flour
- 1 teaspoon baking powder
- 1 teaspoon sea salt
- ¾ cup fat-free milk
- 2 egg whites
- 2 teaspoons honey
- ½ CUP YOGURT CHERRY
- 2 tbsp canola oil
- Spray with canola oil

Preheat oven to 400°F. Combine dry ingredients in a large mixing basin. Combine wet ingredients in a smaller mixing dish. Mix wet ingredients into dry ones until thoroughly mixed. Spray an 8" square pan with canola oil spray and pour in the bread batter. Bake for approximately 20 minutes, or until done, in a preheated oven.

Makes one loaf

Bread with Garlic

I used to make garlic bread with plenty of butter and oil, but this is a better version of that bread. It's straightforward and effective.

- 1 baguette (whole grain)
- 1/4 cup extra virgin olive oil
- 4 minced garlic cloves
- Seasoned with salt & pepper

Preheat the oven to 400°F. Cut the bread lengthwise along the middle. Using a 4-inch segment cutter, cut the bread into 4-inch segments. Combine the olive oil and garlic. Lightly brush with olive oil and garlic. Season with salt and pepper to taste. Place immediately on the rack in the oven for 5 minutes, or until the bread is somewhat crispy.

Serves 5-6

Whole Wheat Bread, Plain

This bread has a lovely crisp crust and is great for sandwiches or toast in the morning.

- 1 pound active dry yeast

- 1 to 2 cup water (110-115 degrees F.)
- 3/4 cup whole wheat white flour
- 1 teaspoon sea salt
- 1 teaspoon honey
- ½ cup fat-free milk (110-115 degrees F.)
- 2 tbsp canola oil
- Dusted with flour
- Spray with canola oil

Allow yeast to dissolve in ½ cups of warm water for 10 minutes.

In a large mixing basin, add the flour and salt; whisk to thoroughly incorporate the ingredients. Next, mix in the honey, milk, yeast mixture, and oil until all ingredients are combined. The dough will be lumpy and uneven. If required, add the remaining water (dough should not be sticky.)

Turn the dough out onto a clean, dry, floured surface and knead for 5 minutes or until smooth. Cover with plastic wrap and place in a greased basin. Allow coming to a boil in a

Warm it in a warm place for approximately an hour or until it doubles in size.

Preheat the oven to 375°F. Punch the dough down and re-roll it out onto the working area. Roll up the dough and put it in a 9 x 5 loaf pan coated with canola oil spray. Allow rising until it doubles in size again (about 1 hour).

Bake for 30 minutes in a preheated oven. Remove the bread from the oven and gently remove it from the pan. Allow cooling on a rack.

Makes one loaf

Garlic Flatbread That Isn't So Flat

These tiny bread are perfect for sandwiches or dips and are best served warm and toasty straight off the grill.

- 1 pound active dry yeast
- 1 cup of water (110-115 degrees F.)
- 4 cups whole wheat flour, white
- ½ cup nonfat milk, room temperature
- 2 egg whites
- 3 tbsp. unrefined brown sugar
- 1 teaspoon sea salt
- 4 minced garlic cloves
- ½ cup fat-free milk (110-115 degrees F.)
- 1/4 cup extra-virgin olive oil
- Dusted with flour
- Spray with canola oil
- Seasoned with salt & pepper

Allow yeast to dissolve in a small dish of water for 10 minutes.

In a large mixing bowl, combine the flour, milk, egg whites, sugar, and salt. Mix in the yeast mixture until a soft dough forms. Turn out of the basin and knead for 5 minutes on a lightly floured surface or until smooth.

Spray a large mixing bowl with canola oil spray and add the dough. Allow the dough to rise until it doubles in bulk, then cover with plastic wrap.

Punch down the dough and knead in 3 garlic cloves. Divide the mixture into ½ equal parts and shape it into ½ tiny balls. Spray a cookie sheet with canola oil spray and arrange the balls on it. Cover with plastic wrap and set aside to double in size.

Combine the remaining garlic with olive oil.

Preheat the grill or skillet to medium heat.

Roll each dough ball out into a 5-inch circle with a rolling pin once it has risen a second time.

Cook for 2-3 minutes, or until the dough puffs up, on the grill or griddle. Brush the uncooked side of the dough with garlic olive oil before turning it over. Brush the cooked side with olive oil and cook for another 2-3 minutes, or until done. Cook the rest of the dough in the same way. Serve fresh off the grill for the best flavour! Season with salt and pepper to taste.

This recipe yields 12 flatbreads.

Bread with Herbs

Because it is yeast bread, it requires a bit more effort and time to make, but it is well worth the time and difficulty. Herbs, both dried and fresh, are high in antioxidants, which may come as a surprise.

- 1 pound active dry yeast
- ¼ cup of water (110-115 degrees F.)
- 1 tbsp. raw brown sugar
- ½ cup scalded and room temperature nonfat milk
- ½ cup extra-virgin olive oil or canola oil
- 1 teaspoon sea salt
- 1 beaten egg white

- 4½ -5 cup whole wheat white flour
- 1 garlic clove, minced
- ½ tsp black pepper
- 1 tsp. ground sage
- 1 teaspoon fresh thyme, diced
- 1 teaspoon fresh rosemary, chopped
- 1 tablespoon finely chopped
- Parsley, flat-leaf
- Dusted with flour
- Spray with canola oil

Preheat the oven to 375°F. Allow yeast to dissolve in warm water for 10 minutes.

Add the sugar, milk, oil, salt, egg white, and 2 cups of flour to the yeast mixture. Cover with plastic wrap after thoroughly mixing with a big spoon. The dough will be a little sloppy. Allow rising in a warm area for approximately 1 hour or until bubbly.

To the dough, add garlic, pepper, and all of the herbs. Add the remaining flour until the dough is smooth. Depending on your altitude, you may need a bit less or a little more flour. Place the dough on a clean, dry, and floured board. Knead for approximately 10 minutes, or until all of the ingredients are combined into a smooth dough. Form into a big ball. Place the dough ball in a large, canola oil-sprayed basin, cover with plastic wrap, and let rise for 1 hour, or until doubled.

Grease a 9-inch loaf pan thoroughly with canola oil spray.

Punch down the dough and put it in an oiled loaf pan. Allow rising until doubled again, approximately 1 hour. Bake in a preheated oven for 40 minutes or until done. Remove bread from the pan (carefully, the pan will be hot) and cool on a rack.

Makes one loaf

Pumpkin Bread with Oatmeal Topping

Pumpkin is high in beta-carotene, an essential antioxidant; a recent study suggests that eating foods high in beta-carotene may decrease the chance of getting some kinds of cancer. Plus, the aroma of pumpkin bread baking is always a pleasant one in the kitchen.

- ½ cup whole wheat white flour
- ¼ cup unrefined brown sugar
- ¼ cup quick-cooking oats
- 2 tablespoons baking soda
- ½ teaspoon ground cinnamon
- ½ teaspoon ground nutmeg
- ½ teaspoon ground cloves
- ½ teaspoon of salt
- ½ cup fat-free milk
- 1 teaspoon fresh lemon juice
- 1 cup plain canned pumpkin
- 2 egg whites
- ¼ cup applesauce, unsweetened
- ¼ cup of canola oil

- ¼ cup raisin

- Spray with canola oil

- ½ cup walnuts, chopped

Preheat the oven to 350°F and coat a 9-inch loaf pan with canola oil spray.

To create fake buttermilk, add lemon juice to the milk.

In a small mixing basin, combine the dry ingredients.

Mix wet ingredients in a larger mixing basin until thoroughly combined.

Stir together the dry and wet ingredients until well combined, then fold in the walnuts and raisins.

Pour into the loaf pan that has been prepared.

Sprinkle the Oatmeal Topping over the top of the loaf and lightly press it in—Bake for 1 hour in a preheated oven or until golden brown.

This recipe makes 1 loaf.

Topping for Oatmeal

- 1 tsp. canola oil

- 1 tsp brown sugar, raw

- ¼ cup quick-cooking oats

- 1 teaspoon ground cinnamon

- ½ tsp ground cloves

Combine all of the ingredients in a mixing bowl and stir until well combined.

Oatmeal Topping on Sweet Potato Bread

Sweet potatoes are high in complex carbs, low in calories, and high in fibre; they have been proven to help prevent cancer and heart disease, and a four-ounce serving provides half of the recommended daily intake of Vitamin C.

- 1 pound active dry yeast
- ¼ cup of water (110-115 degrees F.)
- ½ cup apple juice, unsweetened
- ¼ cup cooked and mashed sweet potato
- 2 cups whole wheat white flour
- ¼ cup chopped walnuts
- 1 teaspoon sea salt
- Spray with canola oil

Preheat oven to 350°F. Dissolve yeast in warm water and set aside for 10 minutes.

In a large mixing bowl, combine all ingredients, including the yeast mixture, except the walnuts and ¼ cups whole wheat flour (for kneading). Mix well until dough forms. Place dough on a smooth, floured surface and knead for about 10 minutes, adding the remaining ¼ cups of flour as needed until the dough is smooth and not sticky.

Spray a 9 5 loaf pan with canola oil spray. Punch the dough down, remove from the bowl, and shape it into a consistent loaf. Cover with plastic wrap and rise again in a warm location for approximately an hour or until dough doubles.

Sprinkle the Oatmeal Topping and walnuts over the dough and gently press the topping into the top of the dough. Bake the bread for 30-35 minutes, or until golden brown.

Makes one loaf

Blueberry Muffins Made with Whole Wheat

Blueberries are a nutritional powerhouse in a tiny colourful package! In addition, blueberries include natural chemicals that may help prevent cancer and cognitive loss.

2 cups whole wheat white flour

- 1 teaspoon baking powder
- ½ teaspoon of salt
- 2 tbsp. unrefined brown sugar
- 1 lemon's zest
- 1 lemon juice
- ¼ cup milk
- ½ cup nonfat plain yoghurt
- 1 ripe banana, peeled and mashed
- 2 egg whites
- ¼ cup of canola oil
- 1 cup fresh or frozen blueberries
- Spray with canola oil

Preheat the oven to 350°F. Combine the dry ingredients in a large mixing bowl. Add the lemon zest to the dry ingredients, then add the lemon juice to the milk to create fake buttermilk.

In a separate bowl, whisk together the wet ingredients. Stir liquid ingredients into dry ingredients and mix well. Gently fold in the blueberries. Spray a 12-muffin pan with canola oil spray and bake in a preheated oven for 20 to 25 minutes, or until golden.

12 muffins are produced.

Irish Soda Bread (Whole Wheat)

This delicious, chewy bread goes well with soups or stews on a cold autumn or winter night.

- 3 cups whole wheat white flour
- 1 cup unbleached all-purpose flour
- 1 teaspoon sea salt
- 2 tsp baking powder
- 2 tbsp cream of tartar
- 1 tbsp. raw brown sugar
- 1½ cup skim milk
- 1 tablespoon of vinegar
- 2 teaspoons olive oil
- Dusted with flour

Preheat oven to 375°F. Combine all dry ingredients in a mixing bowl. Make faux buttermilk by stirring vinegar into skim milk. Pour faux buttermilk into a dry mixture. Add oil. Mix until dough is soft and pliable, adding more milk as needed. The dough should be moist but not sticky. Shape into a flat circle (about 2 inches thick) on a lightly floured surface.

Makes one loaf

Pita Bread (Whole Wheat)

If you have the time, these bread are enjoyable to prepare. Also, if you have kids, what could be better than baking bread with tiny pockets? It's a fast and simple bread recipe that doesn't include any preservatives or harmful oils you may find in store-bought bread. Pitas freeze well, so prepare a few batches and have them on hand for dipping or a fast lunch!

- 1 cup plus 2 tbsp water (110-115 degrees F.)
- 1 pound active dry yeast
- 1 tbsp. raw brown sugar
- 1 cup white unbleached flour
- 2 cups whole wheat white flour
- ½ teaspoons of salt
- 1 teaspoon olive oil
- Dusted with flour
- Spray with canola oil

Allow yeast and sugar to dissolve in a small dish of warm water for 10 minutes.

In a large mixing bowl, combine the flours and salt, then add the yeast mixture and olive oil. Stir until the flour and liquid combine to form a wet dough.

Spray a clean, dry surface with canola oil spray and place the dough on it. To prevent dough from sticking to your hands, spritz them with canola oil spray. Knead the dough for 5 minutes, or until it's smooth and not sticky to the touch. If required, add a little more flour.

Spray a large mixing bowl with canola oil spray and add the dough. Cover and set aside in a warm location for approximately 1 hour, or until the dough has doubled. Preheat the oven to 450°F while the dough is rising.

Punch the dough down and divide it into 8 equal pieces. Roll out each piece into 6-inch circles on a floured surface.

Spray a baking sheet with canola oil and arrange the rounds on it. Preheat the oven to 350°F and bake for 6 minutes, or until the dough puffs. Remove from the oven and wrap in a clean, dry towel to keep moist and tender. To release the air in the pocket, gently press down on the towel. When they're cold enough to handle, cut them in half and fill the pocket. To keep them wet, place them in a food storage bag.

This recipe yields 8 pitas.

Bread with Zucchini

Zucchini is rich in Vitamins A and C, both of which are potent antioxidants. Consumption of zucchini has also been shown in labs to be helpful in the battle against lung cancer. Aside from that, zucchini bread is a true American staple! This whole wheat version is reduced in fat and contains a little honey rather than a big white sugar.

- 2 cups whole wheat white flour
- ½ cup finely shredded and packed zucchini
- ½ cup applesauce, unsweetened
- 2 egg whites
- ¼ cup of canola oil
- 3 tbsp honey
- 1 tsp vanilla extract
- 1 tsp. baking soda

- 1 tsp. baking powder
- ¼ teaspoon cinnamon
- 1 teaspoon ground nutmeg
- ½ tsp ground cloves
- ½ teaspoon of salt
- ½ cup walnuts, chopped
- ½ cup raisin
- Spray with canola oil
- Preheat the oven to 350°F.

Combine the wet ingredients in a large mixing basin.

In a separate large mixing bowl, add the dry ingredients.

Mix the wet and dry ingredients well. Mix in the nuts and raisins.

Pour the batter into a 9 x 5 loaf pan that has been coated with canola oil.

Bake for 1 hour, or until done, in a preheated oven.

Remove the bread from the oven and place it on a wire rack to cool.

Makes one loaf

Bread with Cinnamon and Raisins

Cinnamon is a spice that most of us keep in our cabinets, and it has recently been proven in laboratory tests to both prevent the development and spread of cancer. That's a lot of potential from a single spice.

- 2 cups whole wheat white flour

- ¼ cup unrefined brown sugar
- ½ teaspoon of salt
- 1 teaspoon baking powder
- 1 teaspoon ground cinnamon
- ½ teaspoon ground nutmeg
- 1 tablespoon of vinegar
- 1 ¼ non-fat milk
- ONE EGG
- 2 tbsp canola oil
- ½ cup raisin
- ½ cup walnuts, chopped
- Spray with canola oil
- Preheat the oven to 350°F.

In a large mixing basin, whisk together the flour, sugar, salt, baking powder, cinnamon, and nutmeg. To create fake buttermilk, add vinegar to the milk. In a small mixing dish, combine the milk, egg, and oil.

Stir the liquid mixture into the dry ingredients until thoroughly combined. Add the raisins and ¼ cup walnuts and mix well.

Coat a 9-inch loaf pan with canola oil spray. Fill the loaf pan halfway with batter. Sprinkle the top of the batter with the remaining ¼ cups of chopped walnuts. Lightly press the walnuts into the batter's surface. Bake for 35 minutes or until the bread tests are done. Allow the bread to cool on a wire rack before removing it from the pan.

Note: For the topping, ¼ cups chopped Healthy Trail Mix may be used for the final ¼ cup chopped walnuts.

Makes one loaf

SANDWICHES

Panini with Roasted Vegetables

Sometimes all you want to do is put something between two slices of bread and eat it. It's not that having a sandwich is a bad thing; it's what we've been used to playing between those two slices of bread that's the issue. Meats and fat-laden spreads are the typical culprits, with lunchmeat being the major offender. According to the American Institute for Cancer Research and The World Cancer Research Fund's Second Expert Report, processed meats are among the worst foods we may consume while attempting to prevent cancer.

You may still enjoy a sandwich while being healthy; just select the appropriate stuff to place between those two pieces of whole-grain bread! Serve Roasted Vegetable Panini, for example, at your next party and see if there are any complaints.

Fries and cheeseburger

A vegetarian buddy once told me, "I miss the burger experience." Unfortunately, you won't be able to with them! Burger Nights are a favourite in my home. Although the burgers are delicious, the true pleasure on burger nights is the excellent fries that come with them.

- Burgers with Mushrooms and Cheese
- 2 whole-grain buns
- 2 Veggie Mushroom Burgers
- 2 cheese slices (part-skim mozzarella, veggie, or soy)
- Spray with canola oil

Cook the burgers in a pan coated with canola oil according to the package instructions, adding a slice of cheese to each patty for the final minute of cooking. Serve with handmade fries and your choices of burger toppings, such as avocado, grilled onions, hearty greens, or tomatoes.

Fries

- 1 big russet potato, peeled
- 1 peeled big sweet potato or yam
- 2 teaspoons olive oil
- Seasoned with salt & pepper
- Garlic granules
- Spray with canola oil

Preheat the oven to 450°F. Microwave the potatoes halfway through, piercing them with a fork. Microwave durations vary; you don't want the potatoes completely cooked, just softened. The cooking time in the oven will be reduced as a result. Allow the potatoes to cool once they have been microwaved.

Cut the potatoes into French fry-sized chunks. Drizzle olive oil over the cut potatoes in a bowl. Season with salt, pepper, and garlic to taste. Combine thoroughly. Place the potatoes on a cookie sheet coated with canola oil, flattening them out. Bake for 15-30 minutes, flipping potatoes with a spatula every 5 minutes or so to keep them from burning. They're ready to eat when they're brown and crispy!

Serves 2

Wraps made from lavash

This is a tasty sandwich that is also healthy for you! Beans are a wonder food, and sprouts have been proven in tests to help prevent some malignancies.

- 1 whole-wheat lavash (½-inch square)

- ½ cup hummus
- ½ cup seeded and sliced cucumber
- 1 small sliced onion
- 1 medium seeded and sliced tomato
- 1 cup of sprouts (any kind will do)
- ¼ cup carrots, shredded
- ¼ cup chopped red pepper
- a quarter teaspoon cumin
- ¼ cup fresh cilantro, chopped
- Seasoned with salt & pepper

Distribute the Hummus equally over the lavash. Spread the remaining ingredients equally over the Hummus. Roll the lavash into a long log and cut it in half. Season with salt and pepper to taste. Serve chilled.

Serves 2

Burgers with Portobello Mushrooms

Marinated portobello mushrooms are a tasty alternative to hamburgers. They are tasty and meaty, low in fat, rich in fibre, and have been shown to have anti-cancer effects. This is a tasty alternative to a summertime grilled classic.

4 portobello mushroom caps, big

½ cup balsamic vinaigrette

¼ cup olive oil, extra-virgin

1 minced garlic clove

2 tbsp fresh basil, chopped

2 tbsp flat-leaf parsley, chopped

4 part-skim mozzarella, vegetarian, or soy cheese slices

4 hamburger buns (whole wheat)

Place all of the ingredients (excluding the cheese and buns) in a quart-size plastic food storage bag and seal tightly. Shake vigorously until well combined. Place the bag in the refrigerator to marinate for at least 4 hours or until the mushrooms are plump.

Place the contents of the bag on a hot grill or in a skillet. Cook for about 5 minutes on each side. During the final few minutes of cooking, sprinkle cheese on top of the mushroom. Serve on a whole wheat bun with lettuce, tomato, pickles, and all of your favourite burger toppings.

Serves 4

Burgers with Mushrooms and Veggies

These vegetarian burgers are simple to prepare and delicious. They are much healthier than store-bought alternatives, and there is no risk of carcinogens when grilled. Make a double batch and keep it in the freezer for a quick grill-it-on-the-grill supper.

You'll never miss the meat if you get inventive with your toppings. Isn't that what makes a burger wonderful in the first place? So instead of lettuce, try avocado, sweet or spicy peppers, or arugula. Your creativity only limits your topping options!

- 2 teaspoons olive oil
- 1 pound diced mushrooms
- ½ medium diced onion
- 2 minced garlic cloves

- ½ cup oats, rolled
- ½ CUP BREAD CRUST (preferably Panko)
- ½ cup grated cheese (part-skim mozzarella, veggie, or soy)
- 1 EGG
- 1 tablespoon dried onion
- ½ tsp celery salt
- ¼ tsp. paprika
- ¼ tsp cracked black pepper
- ¼ tsp celery seed
- ¼ cup flat-leaf parsley, chopped
- Spray with canola oil

Sauté the onions, garlic, and mushrooms in olive oil for approximately 5 minutes, or until the onions are tender and the mushrooms have lost all of their water. Set aside until the surface is cold enough to touch.

Combine all of the remaining ingredients, then add the sautéed onions, garlic, and mushrooms.

Stir until all of the ingredients are thoroughly incorporated, and the consistency resembles ground beef. Form the mixture into four patties. Cook each patty in a pan sprayed with canola oil spray until the burgers are done (about 5 minutes on each side). When flipping the burgers, take caution since they are a bit crumbly and not as compressed as a meat burger.

This recipe yields 4 burgers.

Panini with Onion and Pepper

I've always like an Italian pepper sandwich, and this is a wonderful, simple panini recipe. Quick and simple, but delicious and nutritious!

- ¼ cup extra virgin olive oil
- 1 big chopped onion
- 1 big seeded and sliced green pepper
- 1 big seeded and sliced red pepper
- 1 minced garlic clove
- ½ oz. whole wheat baguette
- 6 basil leaves, fresh
- 2 cheese slices (part-skim mozzarella, veggie, or soy)
- Spray with canola oil
- Seasoned with salt & pepper

That's fantastic if you have a panini grill. If you don't have one, wrap an average brick in aluminium foil and use it to compress your panini.

2 tablespoons olive oil, heated in a large pan over medium heat Combine the onions, green pepper, red pepper, and garlic in a mixing bowl. Cook the veggies until they are soft. Season with salt and pepper to taste. Place aside.

Cut the bread into two sandwich pieces, then cut the top of the bread off so that the top and bottom are flat. Brush the remaining olive oil over the top and bottom of the bread, as well as the insides.

Place the bread on a hot grill to gently brown one side. The insides of the sandwiches will be the gently toasted sides. Take the skillet off the heat.

Arrange the veggies on the toasted sides of the two slices of bread. Top with basil, cheese, and bread crusts. Place the sandwiches on a panini grill or a griddle to cook.

Using a panini grill, heat until the sandwich is done according to the panini grill's directions. Place the foil-covered brick on top of the sandwich if using the grill. Cook for 3 minutes, then remove the brick. Flip the sandwich over, replacing the foil-covered brick on top. Cook for a further 3 minutes. Serve immediately and enjoy!

Serves 2

Panini with Roasted Vegetables

What better way to get your vegetables than this?

- ¼ cup balsamic vinaigrette
- ¼ cup olive oil, plus more olive oil for brushing
- 1 minced garlic clove
- 1 medium eggplant, cut into ¼-inch strips lengthwise
- 1 zucchini, cut into ¼-inch strips lengthwise
- 4 moderately sliced portobello mushrooms
- 1 medium onion, peeled and cut into rings
- 1 baguette (whole wheat)
- 1 roasted red pepper, seeded and skinned (or jarred peppers)
- 4 tbsp. Black Olive Tapenade
- 4 part-skim mozzarella, vegetarian, or soy cheese slices
- Spray with canola oil
- Seasoned with salt & pepper

That's fantastic if you have a panini grill. If you don't have one, wrap an average brick in aluminium foil and use it to compress your panini.

Combine the olive oil, balsamic vinegar, garlic, salt, and pepper in a mixing bowl. In a plastic bag, combine the eggplant, zucchini, mushroom, and onion with the oil and vinegar marinade. Refrigerate for 1-3 hours after firmly sealing the bag.

Preheat your panini grill to medium heat. Grill the marinated veggies until grill marks emerge and the vegetables are tender. Set aside after removing from the grill. If you don't have a panini grill, you may grill your vegetables on an outdoor grill or under the broiler, flipping them to cook both sides. Then, take the pan off the heat and put it aside.

Cut the bread into four sandwich pieces, then cut the very top of the bread off so that the top and bottom of the bread are both fats. Brush the top and bottom of the bread, as well as the insides, with olive oil. Place the bread on the grill to gently toast one side. The insides of the sandwiches will be the gently toasted sides. Remove off the grill and set aside.

Place the veggies on the toasted sides of four slices of bread: Tapenade, cheese, and the bread's crust on top. Then, place the sandwiches on a hot panini grill or griddle.

Using a panini grill, heat until the sandwich is done according to the panini grill's directions. If using the grill, put the sandwiches on the canola oil-sprayed skillet, followed by the foil-covered brick. Cook for 3 minutes, then remove the brick. Flip the sandwich over, replacing the foil-covered brick on top. Cook for a further 3 minutes. Serve immediately and enjoy!

Serves 4

Pita Bread Salad

This is a fast and nutritious meal that is also versatile, making it an excellent way to use up salad leftovers. Simply prepare a salad to your taste and put it inside a pita! Simple, fast, and filling.

4 pita bread, sliced in half

- ½ Tbsp. Hummus

- 2 cups chopped hearty greens

- ½ tiny sliced cucumber

- 1 large diced tomato

- ½ cup brown rice, cooked

- 1 big ripe avocado, chopped

- ¼ cup balsamic vinaigrette

- ¼ cup extra virgin olive oil

- 1 pound shredded cheese (part-skim mozzarella, veggie, or soy)

- ¼ cup finely chopped onion

- Seasoned with salt & pepper

Open the pitas and pour 3 tablespoons of the Hummus into each one. In a large mixing basin, combine all of the remaining ingredients. Fill pitas with salad mixture. Shredded cheese on top.

Serves 4

Burgers with salmon

This one fulfils the burger need without the fat of a traditional burger and with the added benefit of omega-3 fatty acids from the salmon. Omega-3 fatty acids have been proven to aid in the prevention of cancer cell development.

- 24 oz. wild salmon

- ¼ cup flat-leaf parsley, chopped
- ¼ cup fresh dill, chopped
- 1 tablespoon chives, finely chopped
- 2 tbsp Dijon mustard
- 2 lemons juice
- 2 minced garlic cloves
- ½ cup grated cheese (part-skim mozzarella, veggie, or soy)
- ½ teaspoon of salt
- ½ teaspoon black pepper
- Spray with olive oil

Finely chop fresh salmon, either by hand or in a food processor, until it resembles ground meat. Mix the salmon with the other ingredients (excluding the olive oil spray) in a large mixing basin. Form the mixture into four patties. Cook for 5 minutes on medium-low heat in a skillet sprayed with olive oil spray. Flip once and cook for another 2 minutes, or until done. Slowly cook the burgers to prevent them from burning. Instead of lettuce and tomato, it was served with a large leaf of mustard for a fun, delicious treat.

Lettuce and tomato! The mustard greens nicely complement the flavour of the Dijon mustard in the burgers.

This recipe yields 4 burgers.

SALADS

Coleslaw with Indian Spices

We think we're eating healthily when we eat a salad, but a lot of the time, the salad dressing has enough fat to sink a ship and may transform salads into a nutritional nightmare!

I have a salad for lunch nearly every day, but I take care to cook it healthily. I dice and chop my veggies at the beginning of the week and then chill them, so they're ready to include in my lunchtime salads, whether I'm dining at home or packing my lunch to go. This does need some preparation, but once you get into the flow of things, it's a piece of cake.

Salads may be a wonderful comfort meal as well as a powerful cancer preventer, but we need to alter how we think about them and what goes into them. They're anything but boring when made with the proper ingredients, and they make a really filling dinner. First and foremost, skip the iceberg lettuce—mainly it's water. Use hearty greens like kale, Swiss chard, and raw spinach instead. Combine it with some darker leaf lettuces, such as baby greens or radicchio. Grill your veggies first, then chill them if desired. Salads may be made in a variety of unique and tasty ways. I've listed a few of my faves here.

Marinated Tomatoes, Arugula, and Mushrooms

The dark green leaves of arugula belong to the cruciferous family, which means that these hardy greens are linked to broccoli, bokchoy, and Brussels sprouts. Some of the most powerful anti-cancer nutrients are found in the cruciferous family of plants. In addition, arugula has a spicy, mustardy taste that makes for an unusual and delicious salad.

- 2 cups chopped tomatoes
- 1/4 cup chopped fresh basil

- 3 minced garlic cloves
- 2 cups arugula, fresh
- 1 cup sliced fresh mushrooms
- 4 tbsp extra virgin olive oil
- 2 tbsp balsamic vinaigrette
- Seasoned with salt & pepper

Combine the tomatoes, basil, olive oil, balsamic vinegar, salt, and pepper in a mixing bowl. Allow marinating for at least 8 hours in the refrigerator. Combine tomatoes, arugula, and mushrooms in a mixing bowl. Serve chilled after thoroughly mixing.

Serves 2

Salad with Asparagus and Tomatoes

Asparagus is not only a delicious seasonal treat, but it also contains a plethora of vitamins and minerals. For example, it contains a lot of glutathione, a chemical is shown in labs to help fight cancers and vitamins A and C. This is an excellent addition to a summer picnic or barbeque.

- 1 pound asparagus, cleaned and trimmed
- ¼ cup olive oil, extra-virgin
- 4 minced garlic cloves
- 2 cups chopped tomatoes
- ¼ cup fresh basil, chopped
- ¼ cup olive oil, extra-virgin

- 2 tbsp balsamic vinaigrette
- Seasoned with salt & pepper

2 tablespoons extra-virgin olive oil, garlic, salt, and pepper Cook on a medium-hot grill or in a 400-degree-F oven. Turn often until the meat is golden, tender, and thoroughly roasted. Allow cooling completely after removing from the grill or oven. Cut into 1-inch cubes. Place aside.

Combine the tomatoes, basil, remaining olive oil, balsamic vinegar, salt, and pepper in a mixing bowl. Combine thoroughly. To the tomato mixture, add the chopped asparagus. Season with salt and pepper to taste. Allow marinating for at least 8 hours in the refrigerator. Serve cold on its own or with other dishes.

a salad composed from dark green leafy vegetables like arugula or spinach

Serves 2

Salad Toppings with Avocado and Tomatoes

This salad is simply guacamole with marinated tomatoes, but you get a very flavorful combination when you combine the two. It's delicious as a salad dressing or as a dip. Whatever method you pick, keep in mind that avocados are rich in the carotenoids lutein and zeaxanthin, both of which are strong antioxidants and have cancer-fighting qualities. Cancer-fighting qualities are also found in onions, tomatoes, and cilantro.

- 2 cups chopped tomatoes
- 1 small minced onion
- 3 minced garlic cloves
- 2 tbsp olive oil (extra-virgin)
- ¼ cup balsamic vinaigrette

- 2 avocados, ripe
- 1 lime's juice
- ¼ cup fresh cilantro, chopped
- Seasoned with salt & pepper

In a mixing bowl, combine the tomatoes, onion, garlic, olive oil, and balsamic vinegar. Season with salt and pepper to taste. Place in the refrigerator for at least 4 hours to marinate. Remove from the refrigerator and drain after marinating.

The avocados should be cut in half. Scoop out the avocado pulp and put it in a bowl.

Well, mash. Combine the lime juice and cilantro in a mixing bowl. Stir in the tomato mixture well. Season with salt and pepper to taste. Serve chilled.

Serves 2-3

Salad with Brown Rice and Curry

This is an intriguing, crunchy salad with the bonus of curry. Curry, walnuts, onions, and whole grains have all been proven to have anti-cancer effects.

- 1 cup of yoghurt cheese
- 1 teaspoon curry powder
- 2 cups brown rice, cooked
- 1 diced green onion
- 1 apple, cored and diced 1 celery stalk, diced
- ¼ cup cranberries, dry

- ¼ cup raisin

- ¼ cup chopped and roasted walnuts

- 1 tbsp. raw brown sugar

- 2 tbsp canola oil

- Seasoned with salt & pepper

Combine the Yogurt, Cheese, and curry powder in a small mixing dish. In a large mixing basin, add all of the other ingredients and well incorporate. Combine with the yoghurt mixture. Combine thoroughly. Serve chilled.

Serves 3-4

Salad with Barley and Vegetables

This lesser-known barley grain is rich in fibre and may help avoid various illnesses, including gallbladder disease, diabetes, and heart issues. Barley also includes antioxidants and phytochemicals, both of which aid in cancer prevention. This is a salad that may be used in a variety of ways. You may very much use whatever veggies, cooked or raw, that you have in your refrigerator.

- 1 small sliced onion

- 1 teaspoon olive oil

- 1 cup uncooked barley

- 3 cups low-fat chicken broth or veggie broth

- 1 small sliced onion

- 1 (16 oz.) can wash and drained garbanzo beans (chickpeas)

- 1 big tomato, diced

- 1 seeded and sliced red pepper
- 1 seeded and sliced green pepper
- 1 small sliced cucumber
- 1 big minced garlic clove
- ¼ cup fresh flat-leaf parsley, chopped
- ¼ cup fresh cilantro, chopped
- ½ cup fresh mint, chopped
- ½ cup celery, chopped
- 1 lime juice
- Seasoned with salt & pepper

Brown onion in oil in a large pan over medium heat until tender. Cook, often stirring, until the barley is slightly golden. Bring the broth to a boil. Reduce the heat to a low simmer, cover the pan, and cook for 45 minutes, or until the barley is soft.

Remove from fire and set aside for 10 minutes until the barley is done to your satisfaction (like mine al dente). Then, place in the refrigerator until completely chilled.

When the barley has cooled, combine it with the other ingredients in a large mixing bowl. Toss thoroughly but gently, then return to the refrigerator for at least 2 hours to cool and let the flavours mingle. Season with salt and pepper to taste.

Serve with Minced Herb Salad Dressing or Creamy Cilantro Salad Dressing.

Serves 3-4

Salad with beets

Most people associate beets with red vegetables, but they also exist in white and yellow varieties (golden). I used golden beets in this recipe, but you may use all red beets if you can't locate them. Red beets may be an effective cancer-fighting food. The pigment that gives beets their deep red colour has been proven to be an efficient cancer fighter in numerous tests.

- 2 big red beets
- 2 hefty golden beets
- ¼ cup fresh basil, chopped
- 3 tbsp extra-virgin olive oil
- 3 tbsp balsamic vinaigrette
- 1 tablespoon Dijon mustard
- ¼ cup chopped walnuts
- 3 cup arugula
- Seasoned with salt & pepper

Preheat the oven to 425 degrees Fahrenheit. Trim the beet tops and roots and thoroughly wash the veggies. Distinguish the golden beets from the red beets. Take two big pieces of aluminium foil and cut them in half (large enough to fold over and seal beets in). Put the red beets in the middle of one piece of foil and the golden beets in the centre of the other. Fold each piece of foil over and seal each package, enclosing the beets firmly. Place the beet packs on a baking sheet and bake for 1 hour or until the beets are tender.

To see whether they're done, poke a beet through the foil with the tip of a sharp knife. The beets are done when the knife slides in easily. Remove the beets from the oven and set them aside to cool while still wrapped in foil. When the beets are cold enough to handle, gently open the foil packages. The skin of the beets will readily peel off if you massage them in cool water. Continue to separate the beets by slicing them and placing the red beets in one small dish and the golden beets in another small bowl.

In a separate large mixing bowl, combine the olive oil, balsamic vinegar, and mustard. Toss in the beets, basil, and walnuts carefully. Season with salt and pepper to taste. Serve on an arugula bed.

Serves 3-4

Salad with Carrots and Raisins

According to the findings of laboratory research, eating carrots helps decrease the chance of developing cancer. Didn't your mother always tell you that they were healthy for you? Carrots contain falcarinol, a natural insecticide that protects them against fungal infections. Carrots are practically the sole source of this molecule in the human diet, and this component has been proven to help prevent cancer when consumed fresh.

- 4 cups shredded carrots
- 1 cup chopped pineapple (fresh or canned)
- 1 big diced apple
- 1 cup of raisins
- ¼ cup chopped walnuts
- ¼ cup chopped celery
- 1 cup of yoghurt cheese (drained in the refrigerator for 24 hours)
- 3 tbsp mayonnaise (light)
- 1 tbsp. raw brown sugar
- Seasoned with salt & pepper

In a large mixing basin, combine all of the ingredients. Chill before serving. This salad is much better if it is allowed to rest in the refrigerator overnight to enable the flavours to mingle.

Serves 3-4

Slaw with Cole Slaw

This is a more conventional slaw than the Indian spicy slaw, but it is also an anti-cancer powerhouse. It includes several anti-cancer nutrients.

Slaw

- 4 cups shredded red cabbage
- 4 cups shredded green cabbage
- 1 medium red onion, thinly sliced
- 2 shredded carrots
- a cup of raisins
- 2 diced apples
- Seasoned with salt & pepper

Sauce

- 3 CUP YOGURT AND CHEESE (drained in the refrigerator for 24 hours)
- 3 tbsp mild olive oil or canola oil
- ¼ cup unrefined brown sugar
- ½ CUP APPLE CUCUMBER VINEGAR

- 1 teaspoon celery seeds
- 1 teaspoon mustard seeds
- 2 minced garlic cloves

In a large mixing basin, combine all of the slaw ingredients. In a small mixing bowl, combine all of the sauce ingredients and whisk until smooth. Mix in the sauce with the slaw ingredients. Season with salt and pepper to taste. Chill before serving. This tastes much better after sitting in the refrigerator overnight to let the flavours blend.

Serves 4-6

Salad with Citrus and Ginger Dressing

Citrus fruits are high in fibre and vitamin C. Citrus intake was linked to a lower risk of most malignancies in Japanese research. This is a lovely salad, perfect for summer or to get you out of the winter blues.

- 2 tangerines
- 1 orange, navel
- 1 grapefruit (pink)
- 1 cup chopped fresh pineapple
- 1 apple, peeled and cut into pieces
- 2 finely chopped chives
- 1/4 cup chopped walnuts
- ½ CUP YOGURT CHERRY
- 1 teaspoon fresh ginger root, grated
- 1 orange's juice

- 1 orange's zest
- 1 teaspoon tahini
- 1 teaspoon honey
- Seasoned with salt & pepper

Remove as much of the white pith from the tangerines, oranges, and grapefruit as possible. Cut into bite-sized pieces. Toss with pineapple, apple, chives, and walnuts in a large mixing basin. To create the ginger dressing, mix Yogurt Cheese, ginger root, orange juice, zest, tahini, and honey in a small bowl. Whisk until smooth. Season with salt and pepper to taste. Pour over the fruit and toss to combine. Chill before serving.

Serves 3 - 4

Salad with Chops

The majority of chopped salads include iceberg lettuce, which is mainly water. This chopped salad is prepared with kale and arugula, two cruciferous vegetables that have been proven to help prevent certain malignancies. A chopped salad has a nice feel to it. This salad is a mash-up of different ingredients. Select the veggies you want. Just make sure to cut them all finely. Enjoy your favourite dressing!

- 1 cup finely chopped kale
- 1 cup finely chopped spinach
- 1 cup coarsely chopped arugula
- ½-pound button mushrooms, coarsely chopped
- 2 big tomatoes, seeded and coarsely chopped
- 1 big carrot, coarsely sliced

- 1 big celery stalk, coarsely sliced
- ½ cup coarsely chopped black olives
- 1 finely sliced red onion
- 1 (15½ ounce) can drain garbanzo beans (chickpeas)
- ¼ cup fresh basil, chopped
- 1 tablespoon fresh oregano, chopped

In a large mixing basin, combine all of the ingredients. To serve, toss with salad dressing and serve chilled.

Serves 3 - 4

Salad with White Eggs

Now and again, I have a craving for a good old-fashioned egg salad sandwich. I can. You'll never miss the yolks since there's so much flavour here! Still, fulfil the desire even if I no longer consume the fat used to come with the old-fashioned version. You'll

- 8 medium eggs
- ¼ cup chopped celery
- ¼ cup chopped onions
- ¼ cup chopped red bell pepper
- ¼ cup chopped tomatoes
- 1 tiny grated carrot
- 1 tbsp mayonnaise dressing (nonfat)
- 3 tbsp. yoghurt cheese

- 1 tablespoon Dijon mustard

- Seasoned with salt & pepper

In a saucepan, combine the eggs. Cover with cold water up to 1 inch above the eggs. Bring to a boil quickly. Simmer for 10 minutes on low heat. Remove the eggs from the fire and rinse them in cold water to halt any further frying. Tap the egg to break the shell, then take off the eggshell.

Remove the yolks and set aside the whites. Prepare the whites by chopping them. Mix the minced egg whites with the other ingredients. Season with salt and pepper to taste. Refrigerate until completely cold. Serve as a sandwich on Plain Ol' Whole Wheat Bread or within a Whole Wheat Pita.

Serves 3 -4

Salad with Fennel

Fennel is a vegetable that is underutilized in the United States, but it should not be. It has a slight licorice taste and is rich in antioxidants. Fennel also includes the phytonutrient component anethole and is rich in fibre. Vitamin C. Anethole has been proven in tests to decrease inflammation and assist prevent the development of cancer. This is a delectable salad delight.

2 fennel bulbs, sliced into ¼-inch strips
- 3 oranges, peeled and sliced into bite-size portions

- 1/4 cup raisin

- 1 finely sliced red onion

- 2 teaspoons olive oil

- 2 tbsp vinegar (red wine)

- 1 tablespoon Dijon mustard

- Seasoned with salt & pepper

To make a vinaigrette, mix the oil, vinegar, mustard, salt, and pepper in a small basin. In a large mixing basin, combine the fennel, oranges, raisins, and onion. Toss the fennel mixture with the vinaigrette to incorporate. Serve chilled.

Serves 2-3

Cole Slaw with Indian Spices

This quadruple threat contains four cancer-fighting ingredients: cabbage, garlic, onions, and turmeric! It also contains omega-3 fatty acids from the oil. Aside from that, it tastes quite nice. Its unique tastes make it an excellent side dish or first-course salad.

Slaw

- 2 cups shredded red cabbage
- 2 cups shredded green cabbage
- 1 little shredded fennel bulb
- 1 finely sliced tiny red onion
- 1 shredded carrot
- ½ cup raisin
- 1 big diced apple
- seasoned with salt & pepper

Sauce

- 1 cup of yoghurt cheese (drained in the refrigerator for 24 hours)

- 2 tbsp mild olive oil or canola oil

- 2 smashed garlic cloves

- 1 tbsp. raw brown sugar

- 1 lemon juice

- 1 tablespoon cumin

- ½ teaspoon turmeric

- 2 teaspoons tahini sauce

- 1 teaspoon celery seed

In a large mixing basin, combine all of the slaw ingredients. In a small mixing bowl, combine all of the sauce ingredients and whisk until smooth. Mix in the sauce with the slaw ingredients. Season with salt and pepper to taste.

Chill before serving. This is much better if it rests in the refrigerator overnight to allow the flavours to blend. It keeps in the refrigerator for a week and still tastes good.

Serves 4 - 6

Mix this cole slaw 50/50 with a garden salad and season with olive oil and vinegar for a really gourmet delight. It makes an excellent lunch salad!

Salad with potatoes

Potatoes aren't all that terrible for you. However, they've received a poor rap due to the harmful methods they're sometimes cooked, as well as the unhealthy toppings that are typically heaped on top. White potatoes contain vitamins, minerals, and phytochemicals. Sweet potatoes are an antioxidant-rich food containing beta-carotene and Vitamin C. So, try this healthier version of an old favourite during your next barbeque or picnic.

- 3 big Idaho potatoes, unpeeled
- 1 peeled big sweet potato, cut into 1-inch cubes
- 1 big sliced onion
- 2 celery stalks, chopped
- 3 big garlic cloves, minced
- 1 seeded and sliced red pepper
- 1 seeded and sliced green pepper
- 1 cup of yoghurt cheese (drained in the refrigerator for 24 hours)
- ¼ cup mayonnaise (light)
- ¼ cup flat-leaf parsley, chopped
- 2 tbsp fresh dill, chopped
- 2 teaspoons olive oil
- 1 tiny jalapeo pepper, seeded and coarsely chopped (optional)
- Seasoned with salt & pepper

Prick the Idaho potatoes with a fork and microwave until soft. Remove from the oven and set aside to cool until you can easily handle them. When the cubes are cold enough to touch, cut them into 1-inch cubes.

Microwave the sweet potato until it is tender. Place aside.

Combine the olive oil, garlic, and onions in a large skillet. Cook, often turning, over medium heat until onions begin to caramelize, approximately 20 minutes. Remove from the heat and set aside to cool.

Combine the potatoes and onions, as well as the other ingredients, in a large mixing basin. Combine thoroughly. Season with salt and pepper to taste. Chill before serving.

Serves 4 - 6

Salad with Kale, Tomatoes, and Avocado

This is a beautiful salad. The flavours blend well in this delicious and nutritious meal.

- 2 cups chopped tomatoes
- 2 smashed garlic cloves
- 2 tbsp. fresh chopped basil
- 2 teaspoons olive oil
- 2 tbsp balsamic vinaigrette
- 1 big bunch of kale, washed and chopped
- 1 chopped ripe avocado
- Seasoned with salt & pepper

Combine the tomatoes, garlic, and basil in a mixing bowl. Combine the olive oil and balsamic vinegar in a mixing bowl. Combine thoroughly. Refrigerate for at least two hours to enable the tomatoes to marinade.

After marinating the tomatoes, combine them with greens and avocado. Combine thoroughly. Season with salt and pepper to taste.

Serves 2

Tomatoes Marinated

Tomatoes contain lycopene, an antioxidant that fights free radicals. This little side dish also includes garlic and olive oil, both of which are anti-cancer nutrients. Aside from being good for you, these tomatoes are very easy to make and provide a rich, savoury taste to any dish. This is great as a side dish, over lettuce, or in a mixed salad. So simple, so tasty, and so healthy for you.

1 pound chopped tomatoes (I prefer to mix and match my kinds to appeal to a wide range of tastes. I use a variety of tomatoes, including cherry, plum, yellow, and black. Mix it up with whatever tomatoes are in season, and don't be afraid to experiment.)

- 1 big garlic clove, smashed
- ¼ cup fresh basil, chopped
- ¼ cup fresh cilantro, chopped
- 2 tbsp balsamic vinaigrette
- 2 tbsp olive oil (extra-virgin)
- Seasoned with salt & pepper

Mix all of the ingredients and place them in the refrigerator for an hour or so before serving to allow the flavours to blend. Before serving, give it another good stir.

Season with salt and pepper to taste.

Serves 2 -3

Salad with Roasted Broccoli

Broccoli is high in vitamins C and A and carotenoids, fibre, calcium, and folate. It's also a good source of phytochemicals, which are being researched for their anti-cancer effects. This salad is nutritious, tasty, and a company favourite.

- 4 cups broccoli florets, cooked till al dente, rinsed and cooled
- ¼ cup extra virgin olive oil
- 3 minced garlic cloves
- 3 tbsp. unsalted toasted sunflower seeds
- 1 diced red onion
- 1 chopped celery stalk
- 1 cup washed and drained canned garbanzo beans (chickpeas)
- 3 tbsp raisins
- Seasoned with salt & pepper

Preheat the oven to 400°F. Coat the broccoli florets with olive oil and chopped garlic in a large mixing basin. Place the florets on a baking sheet or roasting pan and roast, rotating periodically, until cooked to a soft, crisp texture (al dente). Allow cooling after removing from the oven. When the florets have cooled, combine them with the other ingredients in a large mixing bowl. To mix all of the ingredients, toss lightly but thoroughly. Season with salt and pepper to taste. Serve chilled with Creamy Cilantro Dressing over the top.

Serves 4

Salad with Spinach, Mushrooms, and Grilled Onions

This is a variation on a traditional spinach salad (without the bacon!). Grilling the onions beforehand and serving them warm on top of the salad adds a new dimension of flavour to the meal. Spinach is high in vitamins, minerals, and phytonutrients and has been linked to a lower risk of cancer.

- 1 big chopped red onion

- 1 teaspoon olive oil

- 12 ounces baby spinach, cleaned

- 8 ounces sliced white mushrooms

- ¼ cup dried cherries, unsweetened

- ¼ cup chopped and roasted walnuts

Sauté the onions in olive oil in a small pan over low heat. Cook, occasionally stirring until the onions begin to caramelize (about 20 minutes). Remove from the heat. While the onions are frying, combine the spinach, mushrooms, cherries, and walnuts in a large mixing bowl. Dress with Honey Mustard Dressing or Poppy Seed Dressing and toss in the caramelized onions. Serve while the onions are still heated.

Serves 3 – 4

Salad with Roasted Corn

Corn has been around for hundreds of years, and there is a solid reason for this. It's low in saturated fat and cholesterol, and it's high in fibre. Corn comes in various colours, including yellow, white, blue, purple, and red. Grilled corn is an enticing summertime delicacy. Unlike meat, you may grill your vegetables to your heart's content without fear of carcinogens developing.

- 6 big ears husked corn on the cob

- 3 minced garlic cloves

- 2 tbsp fresh cilantro, chopped

- 2 tbsp fresh flat-leaf parsley, chopped

- 1 chopped red pepper

- 1 chopped green pepper
- 1 small peeled, seeded, and chopped cucumber
- 3 chopped green onions
- 1 little sliced red onion
- 1 lemon, juiced and squeezed
- 1 lime, juiced and zipped
- 1 celery stalk, finely chopped
- ½ cup olive oil, extra-virgin
- ¼ cup balsamic vinaigrette
- Spray with olive oil
- Seasoned with salt & pepper

Preheat the grill to high heat. Coat the cobs with olive oil spray until evenly covered.

Place on the preheated grill for 5 minutes, then lower to medium heat. Continue to roast the corn cobs, often flipping until it is beautifully browned and soft.

Allow cooling after removing from the grill. When the roasted corn has cooled, take it from the cob and discard the cobs. Place the corn in a large mixing basin. Combine all of the remaining ingredients in a mixing bowl. Toss until the veggies are evenly covered. Season with salt and pepper to taste. Serve chilled.

Serves 4 -6

Salad with Roasted Vegetables

This is a flexible salad that can be prepared with almost any vegetable combination, although I like root veggies. According to several studies, eating root vegetables may reduce the incidence of kidney cancer. Root vegetables are simple to prepare, inexpensive, and have a long shelf life in the refrigerator. On a cold winter night, this salad makes a hearty dish.

- 2 big carrots, peeled and sliced
- 1 onion, sliced into 1-inch pieces
- 6 quartered red potatoes
- 1 leak that has been cut, washed and chopped
- ½ cup extra-virgin olive oil
- 2 medium peeled beets cut into ½-inch pieces
- 2 fennel bulbs, trimmed and sliced into ½-inch pieces
- 4 minced garlic cloves
- ¼ cup balsamic vinaigrette
- ¼ cup fresh flat-leaf parsley, chopped
- ¼ cup fresh chives, chopped
- Spray with olive oil
- Seasoned with salt & pepper

Preheat the oven to 350 degrees Fahrenheit.

Toss carrots, onion, potatoes, leek, fennel, and garlic in a large mixing dish with ¼ cup olive oil. Place the veggies in the bottom of a roasting pan or big cookie sheet and bake for 30 minutes. Roast for approximately an hour, stirring the veggies with a spatula now and again.

Spread the beets out on a smaller cookie sheet. Spray with olive oil and place on a different rack in the oven (the beets must be cooked separately to prevent the beet colour from spreading). Roast for another hour, stirring the beets with a spatula now and again.

Remove the veggies from the oven when they are soft and put them in a large mixing bowl (do not add the beets). Allow for a 20-minute cooling period. Toss in the remaining olive oil, balsamic vinegar, parsley, and chives until thoroughly combined. Season with salt and pepper to taste. Fold in the beets gently and place in the refrigerator for at least 8 hours to fully cool.

Serve on top of a bed of hearty greens.

Serves 6

Salad with salmon

This is a summertime favourite of mine. You may add whatever toppings you like to the salad, but I prefer to keep it simple to shine through the flavours of the salmon and salad dressing.

Salmon is rich in omega-3 fatty acids, and studies have indicated that omega-3s decrease inflammation and may lessen the risk of cancer. Cruciferous plants have anti-cancer qualities as well, and arugula is one of them.

- 4 (4 ounces) wild salmon fillets
- ½ teaspoon garlic granules
- Seasoned with salt & pepper
- 3 ounces arugula
- 2 cups baby spinach
- 2 medium diced tomatoes
- ½ cucumber, thinly sliced

- 6 finely sliced fresh basil leaves
- ½ cup pitted black olives
- Salad Dressing with Honey Mustard
- Spray with olive oil

Cooking fish on high heat, like cooking meats, may be carcinogenic. Therefore the key is to cook it slowly.

Cooking the fish in foil over low heat is recommended.

Preheat the grill or oven to 300 degrees F.

The fish fillets should be well washed and sprayed with olive oil spray. Season the fish with salt and pepper, then top with the granulated garlic. Wrap the fish in foil (individually or in groups) and cook it on the grill or in the oven. Cook for 10-15 minutes, depending on the size of the fillet.

While the fish is cooking, combine the arugula, baby greens, tomatoes, cucumbers, basil, and olives in a large mixing dish. Toss with Honey Mustard Dressing until thoroughly combined. Season with salt and pepper to taste. Distribute salads evenly among four big plates.

When the fish is done, take it from the foil and place it on different salads.

Serve with a slice of crusty Garlic Bread.

Serves 4

PIZZAS

Pizza with Garlic Salad

Pizza is one of my favourite foods. They are very flexible, and your only limitation is your creativity! I've included a recipe for whole wheat pizza dough, which is simple to prepare and stores nicely. I have a couple of dough balls frozen and ready to defrost for a fast and simple supper. You may also use store-bought pizza dough if it is prepared with nutritional components. It may not be simple since most commercial pizza doughs are produced with white flour, sugar, and hydrogenated oils, all of which you want to avoid. You're far better off preparing your batches and freezing them for later use.

Although I create my pizza sauce, if you're in a hurry, you may use a store-bought sauce instead. Any vegetarian, low-fat pizza or spaghetti sauce would suffice. However, if you have the time, homemade is much superior and only takes around 10-15 minutes to make. I've provided my tried-and-true recipe.

I like making pizzas on the barbecue. If you have one, you'll notice that it helps keep the kitchen's clutter to a minimum. It's a lot of fun to cook this way, plus you can use your grill without worrying about carcinogens! If you don't have a grill, you can bake them instead. I use a pizza paddle to quickly transfer my pizzas into and out of the oven, but if you don't have one, you may put the dough on a cooling rack and place the cooling rack straight into the oven or grill.

Pizzas may be a healthy and delicious addition to your diet if you think outside the pepperoni and cheese box. This is a fantastic way to get your vegetables. I've included a few of my favourite recipes, but the options are limitless.!

Pizza Crust Made with Whole Wheat

- 2 packages active dry yeast

- ¾ cup of water (110-115 F.)

- 3½ cup whole wheat white flour
- 2 tsp. raw brown sugar
- ¾ cup soy or nonfat milk (110-115 F.)
- 1 teaspoon sea salt
- 1 teaspoon olive oil
- Dusting with whole wheat flour
- Rolling out a ½-inch circle with cornmeal
- Spray with olive oil

With a small dish, dissolve the yeast in water. Allow for a 10-minute resting period.

In a mixing dish, combine the flour, raw brown sugar, and salt (you can use a mixer with a dough hook, or do it the old fashioned way, by hand). While mixing, gradually add the milk, yeast, and oil until the dough forms a ball.

Sprinkle flour on the table and set the dough in the work area. Knead the dough for approximately five minutes or until it is smooth. Spray olive oil spray into a large mixing basin. Locate the dough in a bowl, cover with plastic wrap, set it aside in a warm place for approximately an hour or until it has doubled in size. Allow dough to rise for another 30 minutes after punching it down.

Divide the dough into four equal halves. Each will provide a 12" pizza. Cornmeal should be sprinkled on your work surface. Roll out the dough and stretch it into a 12-inch circle. If you have a pizza paddle, dust it with cornmeal before transferring the rolled out dough to it, or put the pizza dough on a cooling rack. You're all set to start filling it with the good things!

This recipe yields four (12-inch) crusts.

Sauce for Pizza

Remember that tomatoes, garlic, and basil have all been proven to reduce the risk of some malignancies.

- 6 medium diced tomatoes
- 1 big garlic clove, minced
- ¼ cup fresh basil, chopped
- ½ tsp dried oregano
- 1 tomato sauce
- 1 tsp brown sugar, raw
- Seasoned with salt & pepper
- Spray with olive oil

Spray an olive oil spray onto a skillet. Toss in the tomatoes and garlic. Simmer on low heat until the water in the tomatoes evaporates. Cook for 5 minutes after adding the other ingredients. Place aside.

Four (12-inch) pizzas are accommodated.

Pizza with Garlic Salad

Who would think to put salad on their pizza? I certainly would! This pizza is made using a simple mixed salad recipe, but feel free to be creative and alter it to your liking.

- 1 pizza crust made from whole wheat
- 3 tbsp olive oil
- 3 garlic cloves, chopped
- 1 medium sliced onion

- 2 tbsp. grated low-fat cheese
- The parmesan cheese
- 1/4 cup grated cheese (part-skim mozzarella, veggie, or soy)
- Dusting with cornmeal
- 1 cup arugula leaves
- 1 cup salad greens (mixed)
- 2 chopped tomatoes
- ½ cucumber, thinly sliced
- ¼ cup fresh basil, chopped
- 3 tbsp olive oil
- 3 tbsp balsamic vinaigrette
- seasoned with salt & pepper

Preheat the oven to 400°F. In a small saucepan, heat 1 tablespoon olive oil and the onion.

Medium-high heat in a skillet. Cook until the onion has become transparent. Set aside to cool after stirring in the garlic.

Sprinkle some cornmeal on a pizza paddle. Place the rolled out pizza dough onto the paddle or a cooling rack at least as big as the rolled out dough. Slide the dough straight onto the oven rack in the middle of the prepared oven, or put the cooling rack in the centre of the preheated oven using the paddle. Cook for 3 minutes or until the dough is somewhat firm. Once the toppings are on the pizza, you may simply take it off the paddle or cooling rack.

When the dough is somewhat hard, gently take it from the oven with a spatula or remove the cooling rack. Do not switch off the oven. Brush the remaining olive oil over the dough and evenly distribute the garlic/onion mixture, leaving a 12-inch perimeter. Top with the two kinds of cheese.

Return the pizza to the oven. Cook for 7-10 minutes longer, or until the crust is crisp and the cheese has melted. Check-in regularly. Toss greens, tomatoes, cucumber, and basil in a medium bowl as the pizza cooks. Dress the salad with olive oil and vinegar. Season with salt and pepper to taste.

Remove the pizza from the oven and top with the salad. Use a pizza cutter or a big knife to cut the pizza.

Serves 2

Pizza with Grilled Asparagus and Mushrooms

This is an intriguing mix and a summertime favourite of mine when asparagus is in season. You are free to use your creativity here. The variety of vegetables available is almost limitless.

- 1 pizza crust made from whole wheat
- 1 asparagus bunch, cut into 1-inch pieces
- 8 ounces sliced fresh mushrooms
- 2 teaspoons olive oil
- Seasoned with salt & pepper
- 4 big fresh basil leaves, chopped
- ½ CUP PIZZA SUGAR
- a quarter-cup of shredded cheese (part-skim mozzarella, veggie, or soy)
- Dusting with cornmeal

Preheat the oven to 400°F. In a mixing dish, combine the asparagus and mushrooms. Drizzle with olive oil, season with salt and pepper, and toss to cover veggies. Place veggies on a grill pan and cook until done, or place in a skillet over medium heat and cook until done. Take the pan off the heat.

Sprinkle some cornmeal on a pizza paddle. Place the rolled out pizza dough onto the paddle or a cooling rack at least as big as the rolled out dough. Slide the dough straight onto the oven rack using the paddle.

Put the cooling rack in the middle of the preheated oven, or place the cooling rack in the centre of the prepared oven. Cook for 3 minutes or until the dough is somewhat firm.

When the dough is somewhat hard, take it from the oven gently using the paddle or remove the cooling rack. Spoon Pizza Sauce into the middle of the dough and spread it out, leaving a 12-inch perimeter on all sides.

Distribute the veggies and basil equally on top of the pie. Distribute the cheese evenly over the pizza. Return the pizza to the oven. Cook for 7-10 minutes longer, or until the crust is crisp and the cheese has melted. Check regularly to avoid burning. Place on a big platter, slice using a pizza cutter or large knife, and serve!

Serves 2

Pizza with Tomato and Basil

This pizza contains just a few basic ingredients, but it's a hit nevertheless. It's especially good on the grill in the summer when the basil is fresh, and the variety of tomatoes is abundant.

- 1 pizza crust made from whole wheat
- 2 cups cherry tomatoes, halved
- 4 freshly washed and cut basil leaves
- ½ CUP PIZZA SUGAR

- A quarter-cup of shredded cheese (part-skim mozzarella, veggie, or soy)

- Seasoned with salt & pepper

Preheat the oven to 400°F. Sprinkle some cornmeal on a pizza paddle. Place the rolled out pizza dough on the paddle or a cooling rack as least as big as the rolled out dough. Slide the dough straight onto the oven rack in the middle of the prepared oven, or put the cooling rack in the centre of the preheated oven using the paddle. Cook for 3 minutes or until the dough is somewhat firm. Remove the dough from the oven using the pizza paddle or remove the cooling rack when it is somewhat hard. Do not switch off the oven. Spoon Pizza Sauce into the middle of the dough and spread it out, leaving a 12-inch perimeter on all sides. Distribute the tomatoes and basil equally over the sauce. Season with salt and pepper to taste. Distribute the cheese equally over the tomatoes and basil.

Return the pizza to the oven. Cook for 7-10 minutes longer, or until the crust is crisp and the cheese has melted. Check regularly to avoid burning. Slice and serve on a big dish.

Serves 2

Pizza from Mexico

This is a unique take on a traditional meal. It contains all the tastes of Mexican cuisine and the goodness of beans, onions, and tomatoes.

- 1 pizza crust made from whole wheat

- 1 medium sliced red onion

- ¼ cup drained canned sweet corn

- 1 teaspoon olive oil

- ½ (15 oz.) fat-free refried beans

- ¼ cup drained salsa
- ½ can (7 oz.) green chillies
- ½ cup chopped black olives
- 1 cup chopped fresh tomatoes
- ¼ cup fresh cilantro, chopped
- 2 tbsp fresh oregano, chopped
- ¼ -cup of shredded cheese (part-skim mozzarella, veggie, or soy)
- Seasoned with salt & pepper
- To taste, chopped jalapeo (optional)

Preheat the oven to 400°F. Sprinkle some cornmeal on a pizza paddle. Place the rolled out pizza dough on the paddle or a cooling rack as least as big as the rolled out dough. Slide the dough straight onto the oven rack in the middle of the preheated oven, or put the cooling rack in the centre of the oven, using the paddle.

Oven preheated. Cook for 3 minutes or until the dough is somewhat firm.

When the dough is somewhat hard, gently take it from the oven with a spatula or remove the cooling rack. Do not switch off the oven. Place refried beans in the middle of the dough and spread them evenly over the dough, leaving a 12-inch border on all sides. Spread salsa on top of the refried beans, then top with green chillies. Spread sautéed onions and tomatoes evenly on top of the remaining ingredients, followed by olives on top of the pizza. Sprinkle with cilantro and oregano, then top with a layer of cheese, leaving a 12-inch border on all sides.

Return the pizza to the oven. Cook for 7-10 minutes longer, or until the crust is crisp and the cheese has melted. Check regularly to avoid burning. Place on a big platter, cut into slices using a pizza cutter or a large knife, and serve!

Serves 2

Pizza with Pesto

What could be better than pesto and tomatoes? Both contain cancer-fighting qualities and are delicious! Leaving the chunky tomatoes results in a big, full pizza with a delicious bite.

- 1 pizza crust made from whole wheat

- ¼ CUP PESTO SUGAR

- A quarter-cup of shredded cheese (part-skim mozzarella, veggie, or soy).

- 4 plum tomatoes, chopped into 12-inch pieces

- 6 ounces cooked shredded white flesh chicken (optional)

- Spray with canola oil

Preheat the oven to 400°F. Sprinkle some cornmeal on a pizza paddle. Position the rolled-out pizza dough on the paddle or a cooling rack as least as big as the rolled-out dough. Using the paddle, slide the dough straight onto the oven rack in the middle of the preheated oven, or place the cooling rack in the centre of the prepared oven. Cook for 3 minutes or until the dough is somewhat firm. Remove the dough from the oven gently, but do not switch off the oven. Spread pesto sauce evenly over the pizza, leaving a 12-inch perimeter. Distribute tomatoes and shredded chicken (if using) equally on top of pizza, leaving a 1/2 inch boundary around the edge. On top, sprinkle with the cheese. Return the pizza to thc oven. Cook for 7-10 minutes longer, or until the crust is crisp and the cheese has melted. Check-in regularly.

Serves 2

Pizza with Sautéed Peppers and Onions

I used to enjoy an Italian sausage sandwich covered with sautéed onions and peppers when I ate meat. Although Italian sausage is no longer a part of my diet, the flavour of those delicious peppers does not have to be!

- 1 pizza crust made from whole wheat
- ½ julienned green pepper
- ½ julienned red pepper
- ½ julienned yellow pepper
- 1 julienned onion
- 4 fresh basil leaves, chopped
- 1 teaspoon chopped fresh oregano
- 2 teaspoons olive oil
- ½ CUP PIZZA SUGAR
- ¼ -cup of shredded cheese (part-skim mozzarella, veggie, or soy)
- Seasoned with salt & pepper

Preheat the oven to 400°F. In a mixing dish, combine the peppers and onions. Drizzle with olive oil and season with salt and pepper. To coat the veggies, combine all of the ingredients in a large mixing bowl. Cook over medium heat until the vegetables are al dente. Take the pan off the heat.

Sprinkle some cornmeal on a pizza paddle. Place the rolled out pizza dough on the paddle or a cooling rack as least as big as the rolled out dough.

Slide the dough straight onto the oven rack in the middle of the prepared oven, or put the cooling rack in the centre of the preheated oven using the paddle. Cook for 3 minutes or until the dough is somewhat firm.

When the dough is somewhat hard, gently take it from the oven with a spatula or remove the cooling rack. Do not switch off the oven. Spoon Pizza Sauce into the middle of the dough and spread it out, leaving a 12-inch perimeter on all sides. Arrange cooked vegetables equally on top of the sauce, then top with cheese.

Return the pizza to the oven. Cook for 7-10 minutes longer, or until the crust is crisp and the cheese has melted. Check regularly to avoid burning. Place on a big platter, cut into slices using a pizza cutter or a large knife, and serve!

Serves 2

Pizza with Roasted Vegetables

I've selected these veggies, but you may use any vegetables you like.

- 1 pizza crust made from whole wheat
- 5 teaspoons olive oil
- 2 cups broccoli, cut into 1-inch cubes
- 2 cups cauliflower, cut into 1" cubes
- 2 carrots, peeled and cut into 1-inch pieces
- 1 onion, sliced into 1-inch cubes
- 1 big tomato, diced
- Seasoned with salt & pepper
- 2 minced big garlic cloves

- 4 big fresh basil leaves, chopped
- 1 tablespoon chopped fresh oregano
- ¾-cup of shredded cheese (part-skim mozzarella, veggie, or soy)
- 2 tbsp. grated low-fat cheese
- The parmesan cheese
- Dusting with cornmeal

Preheat the oven to 400°F. In a mixing dish, combine the broccoli, cauliflower, carrots, and onion. Drizzle with olive oil, season with salt and pepper, and toss to cover veggies. Place the veggies in a 9 x 13 baking dish and bake for 30 minutes in a preheated oven. Cook for 30 minutes, or until the veggies are al dente. Mix with a big spoon now and then to keep the fire from starting. Take the pan out of the oven.

Sprinkle some cornmeal on a pizza paddle. Place the rolled out pizza dough on the paddle or a cooling rack as least as big as the rolled out dough. Slide the dough straight onto the oven rack in the middle of the prepared oven, or put the cooling rack in the centre of the preheated oven using the paddle. Cook for 3 minutes or until the dough is somewhat firm. Once the toppings are on the pizza, you may simply take it off the paddle or cooling rack. When the dough is somewhat hard, gently take it from the oven with a spatula or remove the cooling rack. Do not switch off the oven.

Combine the garlic and 2 tablespoons olive oil and distribute it over the pizza dough, leaving a 12-inch perimeter. Sprinkle the oregano and basil equally over the dough, followed by the veggies evenly over the herbs and the cheese over the vegetables. Bake for a further 7-10 minutes, or until the crust is crisp and the cheese has melted. Garnish with Parmesan cheese, slice, and serve! Check-in regularly.

Serves 2

CPSIA information can be obtained
at www.ICGtesting.com
Printed in the USA
LVHW051525150623
749768LV00011BA/285